GUIDE TO PSYCHIATRY

Singapore Perspective

16th Revision

GUIDE TO PSYCHIATRY

Singapore Perspective

16th Revision

Chee Kuan Tsee

Institute of Mental Health, Singapore

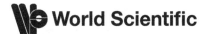
World Scientific

NEW JERSEY · LONDON · SINGAPORE · BEIJING · SHANGHAI · HONG KONG · TAIPEI · CHENNAI · TOKYO

Published by

World Scientific Publishing Co. Pte. Ltd.

5 Toh Tuck Link, Singapore 596224

USA office: 27 Warren Street, Suite 401-402, Hackensack, NJ 07601

UK office: 57 Shelton Street, Covent Garden, London WC2H 9HE

British Library Cataloguing-in-Publication Data
A catalogue record for this book is available from the British Library.

GUIDE TO PSYCHIATRY
Singapore Perspective
16th Revision

For photocopying of material in this volume, please pay a copying fee through the Copyright Clearance Center, Inc., 222 Rosewood Drive, Danvers, MA 01923, USA. In this case permission to photocopy is not required from the publisher.

ISBN 978-981-122-900-8 (hardcover)
ISBN 978-981-123-130-8 (paperback)
ISBN 978-981-122-901-5 (ebook for institutions)
ISBN 978-981-122-902-2 (ebook for individuals)

For any available supplementary material, please visit
https://www.worldscientific.com/worldscibooks/10.1142/12063#t=suppl

Printed in Singapore

Guide to Psychiatry [Singapore Perspective] — (16th Revision)

The current *Guide to Psychiatry — Singapore Perspective* may be considered the 16th edition of the original *Guide to Psychiatry* series, which has been revised and updated every two to three years since the early 1980s. While it was originally written for new doctors posted to Woodbridge Hospital/Institute of Mental Health, its distribution was later extended to general practitioners, psychologists, medical students, allied mental health workers, and other interested readers.

Much of the subject matter derives from five decades of personal clinical experience and some of the thoughts expressed may be unorthodox. The current publication version remains a guide to appreciating psychiatry and the management of local patients. Attempts are made to explain concepts, issues, ambiguities, and principles that are commonly confronted by and confusing to beginners. Analogies are freely used to aid understanding. As mentioned in earlier revisions, this publication does not fulfil the role of a textbook or handbook, of which many have already been written. Nevertheless, this little book can be read over and again as an accessible guide for training psychiatrists, medical doctors and students, and other mental health workers.

Despite the controversies of the DSM 5 and the ICD 11 being far from finalised, these are referred to as much as possible. Regretfully, references are not provided in this book. Any acknowledgement is mentioned in the text itself.

In conclusion, I shall like to express my deep appreciation to Moses Hng Kak Tat for his tremendous help in all aspects of the publication of the book.

Dr. Chee Kuan Tsee
Emeritus Consultant
Institute of Mental Health
Singapore
Email: guidetopsychiatrybook@gmail.com
17 Feb 2020

Reviews

Dr Chee Kuan Tsee can be rightfully said to be the Father of Psychiatry in Singapore. He has trained generations of psychiatrists, all of whom have benefitted from his clear knowledge of psychiatry and are all the better for it. He is deservedly Emeritus Consultant for his many contributions to the specialty. He is always reflecting on many aspects of psychiatry, making the effort to update himself even after retirement. In this respect, he practices what he teaches, which is the hallmark of a great educator.

I remember how he was very strict with case presentations, paying much attention to systematic history gathering, mental state examination, and accurate descriptions of psychopathology. This prevented us from becoming "woolly" in our thinking, which is something psychiatry as a science needs to avoid. At the same time, he constantly encouraged us to acquire in-depth knowledge of our patients' psychosocial background so as to appreciate the impact of their condition on both the individual and his or her family. This showed in his humane approach towards patient care and his practice of the "art of understanding" in psychiatry. All of these are captured in the current revision of his excellent book, *Guide to Psychiatry*.

One of his clinical pearls I appreciate is in the clerking of patients: "the novice should be like a faithful video recorder than an impressionist artist". In the age of electronic documentation, this is particularly noteworthy.

Dr Andrew Peh Lai Huat
MBBS, MMed (Psychiatry), FAMS
Chief, Psychological Medicine
Changi General Hospital

I am privileged to have been taught by Prof Chee as a trainee more than a quarter of a century ago. Observing him at work never failed to awe me. He was sharp and focused during history taking, formulation, and treatment planning, yet warm and empathetic toward his patients. As a mentor, he guided me through the wilderness of my traineeship and early career.

This book is the amalgam of factual information and personal insight that Prof Chee has gleaned through years of practice as a clinician and teacher. It contains the gems of his teaching and practice as well as his personal philosophy and reflections. It serves not only as a clinical guide for the practice of psychiatry in Singapore, but also as a moral and ethical compass.

Concisely written with helpful flow charts and tables, the *Guide to Psychiatry* is an easy read for young trainees and yet thought-provoking for seasoned clinicians. Having reread it many times myself, it has been a reassuring platform for my feet and a light for my path through different eras of my clinical practice.

Dr Liow Pei Hsiang
MBBS, MMed (Psych), FAMS
Senior consultant Psychiatrist
Khoo Teck Puat Hospital

Deeply engaging and highly insightful, Prof Chee's clinician-teacher skills unveil the core of what every psychiatrist's training aims to fulfil. To help bring comfort, encouragement, and healing to the person with mental illness is both an art and a science. Comprehensive and yet concise and compassionate, his conceptual clarity, practical approaches, and creative options shine through these remarkable pages.

I highly recommend this outstanding resource for doctors, psychiatrists, and clinical teachers across geographical and cultural boundaries. Like myself, many have benefited immensely from this God-given, gifted teacher and mentor. He never hesitates to challenge us while showing us true clinical competence plus the meaning and value (not just quality) of life as we navigate through the maze of ever increasing scientific data, changing legal processes, and ethical dilemmas with his sound knowledge, razor-sharp mind, extensive clinical experience, and earnest humility.

Practicing the principles outlined here will ignite your own passion to think through complex clinical, legal, and ethical issues to help patients and families handle social stigma and other devastating consequences of mental illness. With this book, Prof Chee will continue to inspire generations of doctors and mental health professionals to conquer many mountains and remove multiple barriers to recovery.

Dr Arthur Lee Kiat Siong PBM,
MBBS, MMed (Psych), FAMS
International Fellow (American Psychiatric Association)
Dr Art Lee Psych & Counseling Clinic, Gleneagles
Medical Center

It is with immense pleasure and humility that I am able to pen these few lines for the 16th revision of Professor Chee Kuan Tsee's *Guide to Psychiatry*, a most venerable and, I would hasten to add, durable work which has seen the nurturing of many generations of psychiatrists in training, including myself. Speaking as one who has had the unique privilege of being privy to every single edition of Prof Chee's labour of love through the decades, I have no hesitation in stating that *Guide* is the most accessible and concise yet comprehensive introduction to the art and science of clinical psychiatry ever written. As a first-year trainee, the 2nd edition of *Guide* was my constant nocturnal companion on call (and which still sits, incidentally, on the shelf in front of me); close to three decades later as a senior forensic psychiatrist who often has to explain complex psychiatric and psychopathological concepts in our courts of law, I still have regular recourse to the 15th edition of Prof Chee's work as the very best resource that distils with the most practical clarity the principles and practice of clinical psychiatry.

Prof Chee has always been an advocate of lifelong learning; a senior colleague just remarked to me that he has consistently kept himself up to date with the ever burgeoning advances in psychiatry, and this would only be too evident to anyone perusing the pages of his work. Stripped of all verbiage, I am able to state without reservation that but for Prof Chee's unswerving fidelity and dedication to constantly updating *Guide*, I would be a lesser psychiatrist today.

Dr Stephen Phang
Senior Consultant
Dept of Forensic Psychiatry
Institute of Mental Health

Professor Chee has distilled the science and art of psychiatry into an accessible and invaluable guide for psychiatry trainees and other healthcare professionals with an interest in mental health.

What makes this book especially unique are the local nuances that succinctly capture the mental health landscape in Singapore. It is a must-read for all mental health practitioners who practice or intend to practice locally.

Dr Marcus Tan Zhongqiang
Consultant
Geriatric Psychiatry
Institute of Mental Health

The parables are very helpful in relating the challenges of peers. It is one of the more comprehensive handbooks I have seen that covers a wide array of topics ranging from dealing with stigma to understanding clinical terms. I believe anyone who is new to the field of mental health should read it to kickstart their understanding.

Lee Zhong Yi,
Peer Support Specialist,
EPIP, Institute of Mental Health

Contents

Introduction

In **medical disease**, there are physical and/or mental symptoms and typically a recognised aetiology, demonstrable pathology, and predictable course based on biological or physical factors.

In **mental disorder**, there are mental and/or physical symptoms, but one tends to talk of **predisposing**, **precipitating**, and **propagating** factors which can be physical, psychological, or social.

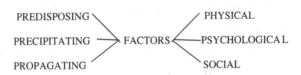

Whether the individual suffers from medical disease or mental disorder, there is complaint of discomfort, distress, disability, or dependency caused by disturbed structure or function. When **subjective experience** is corroborated by **observed behaviour**, an illness is present or considered. It should be appreciated that mental illness is as real and as incapacitating as physical illness.

Nature of Psychiatric Problems

The human person has **physical**, **psychological**, **social**, and **spiritual** attributes that are **inter-related**, **interactive**, and **integrated** in function. In other words, there is inter-relation, interaction, and integration between the **individual** and his **environment**, between his **body** and **mind**, between his **mental functions** and **neural circuits**, and between his **past** and **present life events** and **experiences** (in continuous responses).

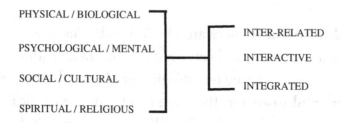

Disturbance in any one aspect would affect the well-being of the rest, causing stress and distress to the individual as a **whole**. Depending on the **proportions** of biological, psychological, social, and spiritual factors or the dominant factor involved, the patient may suffer from an obvious organic disease (e.g., epilepsy, brain infection, dementia), a psychiatric illness (e.g., schizophrenia, depression, paranoid state), a psychosocial reaction (e.g., anxiety, phobia, adjustment disorder), a problem in day-to-day living (e.g., relationship difficulty, domestic crisis, stress in employment), or a religious experience with spiritual struggle.

As a result, there are medical, psychological, sociological, and cultural **theories** and **models** of mental disorders as well as spiritual explanations of morbidity.

Biological/Medical Concept — Pathological Abnormality
Social / Cultural Concept — Statistical Deviation

Psychological/Behavioural Concept—Developmental Impairment
Spiritual / Religious Concept — Supernatural Visitation

However, more commonly the aetiology is **multifactorial**, the complaints are **multifaceted**, and the management is **multidisciplinary**.

Apart from the common **psychotic** symptoms (i.e., hallucinations, delusions, thought disorders, abnormal mood, and anomalous behaviour), psychiatric problems often present with symptoms of aches and pains, breathlessness and giddiness, palpitation and fear, poor concentration and forgetfulness, nervousness, sadness or irritability, insomnia, anorexia or bingeing, weight loss or gain, impotence or loss of libido, social withdrawal, sense of worthlessness or hopelessness, loss of interest, pleasure, energy, apparent laziness, slowness or stupidity, hyperactivity, compulsive or addictive behaviour, and deterioration in work performance. For obvious reasons, it is necessary to exclude any underlying physical disease that could produce both somatic and mental symptoms.

According to the nature of each case, the emphasis may be completely medical, psychological, social, or spiritual. But more often than not, the problem or disorder is **multifactorial in causality** and therefore **multidisciplinary in management** with consideration of predisposing, precipitating, perpetuating, and protective factors. This is all the more so in the developing young and the declining old, whose problems are frequently **multi-axial** in nature. No single theory explains all and no single treatment is comprehensive. It is only practical to be **holistic** (integrating) and **eclectic** (combining).

Size of Psychiatric Problems

Depending on **concepts**, **definitions**, **criteria**, **methodology**, **demographic pattern**, **economic development**, **geographical**

area, **natural disaster**, **migration movement**, **cultural practice**, and **lifestyle**, epidemiological data may vary widely and often be of questionable validity and reliability. Much depends on the quality of resource and research as well as changes that take place during the time frame of studies. Based on reported studies or surveys, the prevalence of "major" psychiatric disorders such as schizophrenia and depression (broadly conceived) is roughly about 0.5–1% and 10% respectively. The prevalence of "minor" psychiatric morbidities like "neurotic" disorders stands at about 15–20%, and mental retardation or intellectual disability of various degrees occurs around 2–3% of the population. These figures are not static and change with time and circumstances. Dementia prevalence would grow with an ageing population while the young are constantly exposed to the danger of abuses, drugs, and the internet. Alcohol dependence and addictive behaviours such as problem gambling and computer games are also a major area of growing concern. About 5–10% of those over 60 years old would suffer from dementia.

The 2016 Singapore Mental Health Study reported that about 1 in 7 people over 18 years old has experienced a mood, anxiety, or alcohol abuse disorder in their lifetime. Major depressive disorder (MDD), alcohol abuse, and obsessive-compulsive disorder (OCD) are the top three mental disorders. MDD is the most common with 1 in 16 persons (6.25%), followed by alcohol abuse with 1 in 24 (4+ %) and OCD with 1 in 28 (3.5+ %). Probably less than 10% of the population suffer from anxiety. About 10% of those over 60 years of age would suffer from dementia, of which around half would be due to cerebral vascular accidents or strokes. Unlike Alzheimer's dementia, vascular causes are more preventable and treatable.

Goldberg and Huxley (1980) studied the **pathway to psychiatric care.** In a community survey of a random population sample of 1,000 (one-year period prevalence, median estimates), 250 were noted to have some complaints. Of these, 230 exhibited illness behaviour and sought help at primary care level and 140 were detected to have conspicuous psychiatric morbidity. Only 17 were referred to a psychiatrist and 6 were eventually admitted to mental hospital. The hospital-based figures therefore represent only the tip of the problem and highlight the importance of primary care service. Nowadays, the emphasis is on reducing hospital beds and improving comprehensive community service.

PATHWAY TO PSYCHIATRIC CARE — GOLDBERG & HUXLEY (1980)
(ONE-YEAR PERIOD PREVALENCE, MEDIAN ESTIMATES)

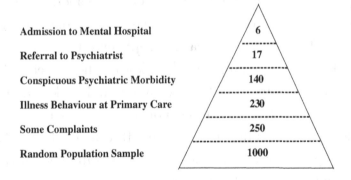

Admission to Mental Hospital	6
Referral to Psychiatrist	17
Conspicuous Psychiatric Morbidity	140
Illness Behaviour at Primary Care	230
Some Complaints	250
Random Population Sample	1000

Problem of Terminology

Psychiatric terminology is still in a flux. Mental disorder is a generic term that covers all the mental conditions that fall within the specialty of psychiatry. In common practice, it includes mental illness, mental retardation (intellectual disability), personality disorder, substance abuse, and sexual deviancy. Mental illness is traditionally divided into psychoses and neuroses. Mental disease is an old term for psychosis or insanity, and disease of the mind is more legal in origin and usage than medical. The "mind" in the Mc'Naghten Rules is used in the ordinary sense of mental faculties of reason, memory, and understanding. Thus, if these faculties are impaired, disease of the mind is present and it matters not whether the aetiology of the impairment is organic or functional, permanent, or transient (**Diplock**).

Concept of Normality

In general, what is "normal" may refer to the **absence of pathology**, a **statistical average**, or an **ideal norm**. There is less controversy when the concept is medical, but when the concept is **psychosocial** and based on **mores** and **norms**, then what is normal or abnormal may vary from one society to another and from one period of time to another. This has implications for therapy because **different aetiological concepts** exist for the same clinical syndrome (e.g., eating disorders, koro). The clinician should be familiar and wary of differences in cultural background, religious belief, political system, economic development, prevalent lifestyle, gender identity, and changing thresholds. For instance, being a virgin after a certain age could be a source of embarrassment if not anxiety and depression in a permissive and promiscuous society. Conversely, in a conservative culture, losing one's virginity out of wedlock may result in guilt, shame, and suicide. However, values can be eroded, lifestyles can be changed, and norms can be imposed upon. In the process, the Asian extended family system and values break down and ironically the therapist now has to learn family therapy from the West, which itself does not appear to sanctify marriage. There is some truth that what is "right" is often defined by "might". But nowadays the catchword is **globalisation**.

It is also important to realise that a **statistical deviant** is not quite the same as a **pathological abnormality**, although one may merge into the other. For instance, it has been said that "he is so bad, he must be mad". The response to this is: "Whatever happens to sin?" It is not always easy to separate variation from morbidity; that is, in mental retardation or intellectual disability, personality disorder(s), and borderline conditions. With the completion of the Human Genome Project, there may be increased "medicalisation" of human anomalies. There is also a tendency to pathologise existential human imperfections and sufferings or habits. For the individual, normality may refer to his/her **premorbid baseline**.

Classification of Mental Disorders

Different countries may adopt **different** national systems of classification of mental disorders. By and large, the Glossary of Mental Disorders (Chapter V) of the World Health Organization's **International Classification of Diseases** 10th Revision (ICD-10), 1992 has been used by governments worldwide for coding and statistical compilations. This would be replaced by ICD-11, Chapter 06, which was provisionally published in 2018 but will probably only be operationally finalised sometime in the near future. ICD provides **prototypic descriptions** of mental disorder for all levels of clinical users. The American Psychiatric Association's (APA) **Diagnostic and Statistical Manual of Mental Disorders** 5th Edition (DSM-5), 2013 continues to provide **criteria sets** of mental disorder favoured by researchers. However, it is neither accepted universally nor even by American psychiatrists themselves. The nomenclature and classification of mental disorders as well as their concepts and descriptions are therefore not universally same or static. In Singapore, the WHO ICD is officially used, although the DSM is also widely referred to professionally and clinically. There is much similarity and compatibility between the two, though differences exist. There are also different versions of ICD-10 for different levels of users (e.g., primary health worker, clinician, researcher). However, in DSM-5 diagnostic classifications, the same criteria and definitions are used for clinical, research, forensic, administrative, educational, and insurance purposes. It avoids theoretical discussions on causes and effects and is a non-axial system. There would be changes as well as harmony in the new revisions of DSM-5 (May 2013) and ICD-11, 2018.

The current WHO ICD-11 [2018] Chapter 06 refers to Mental, Behavioural, or Developmental Disorders. This Chapter has 161 four-character categories and the code range starts with 6A00.

"Mental, behavioural and neurodevelopmental disorders are syndromes characterised by clinically significant disturbances in an individual's cognition, emotional regulation, or behaviour that reflects a dysfunction in the psychological, biological, or developmental processes that underlie mental and behavioural functioning. These disturbances are usually associated with distress or impairment in personal, family, social, educational, occupational, or other important areas of functioning."

Exclusion: Acute stress reaction (QE84)
                    Uncomplicated Bereavement (QE62)
Coded Elsewhere: Sleep wake disorders (7A00-7B2Z)
                    Sexual dysfunction (HA00-HA 6Z)

The chapter contains the following top-level blocks:

* Neurodevelopmental disorders
* Schizophrenia or other primary psychotic disorders
* Catatonia
* Mood disorders
* Anxiety and fear-related disorders
* Obsessive-compulsive or related disorders
* Disorders specifically associated with stress
* Dissociative disorders
* Disorders of bodily distress or bodily experience
* Feeding or eating disorders
* Elimination disorders
* Disorders due to substance use or addictive behaviours
* Impulse control disorders
* Disruptive behaviour or dissocial disorders
* Personality disorders and related traits
* Paraphilic disorders
* Factitious disorders
* Neurocognitive disorders
* Mental or behavioural disorders associated with pregnancy, childbirth, and the peuperium
* Secondary mental or behavioural syndromes associated with disorders or diseases classified elsewhere

The current developments in genetics and neurosciences are probably not yet helpful in the categorisation of mental disorders. In fact, one century ago, **K. Jasper** said while discussing the status of research on the neural correlates of mental disorders that "we only know the end links in the chain of causation from soma to psyche and vice versa, and from both these terminal points we endeavor to advance." In other words, there are still gaps of mutual causative understanding between pathogenesis, pathophysiology, psychosocial factors, and the forms and contents of psychopathology.

Pathogenesis ? ↔ ? Pathophysiology ? ↔ ? Psychopathology ? ↔ ? Psychosocial Factor

(in vice versa of cause or effect)

Hence, the statement remains relevant today and there is still some distance between the terminal points. The US NIMH Research Domain Criteria (RDoC) bridges the gap somewhat between clinical diagnosis and neuroscience.

It is to be reiterated that unlike medical disease, which is diagnosed and treated according to known aetiology, mental disorder is **multifactorial in causality** and **multidisciplinary in management**.

There is constant **inter-relation**, **interaction**, and **integration/dissociation** between:

a) Individual and environment — endogenous and exogenous factors, (e.g., conception, genes, birth, growth, development, family and relationship, work and stress, crisis, climate, disaster, war, persecution and migration, economics and politics)

b) Body/brain and mind — physical systems (organic factors) and psychological systems (mental factors)

c) Mental functions and neural circuits — neurotransmitters and "wiring" (note billions of neurons, trillions of synapses and myriads of circuitries, and 100-odd of neurotransmitters; more complex than computers in functions and dysfunctions)

d) Past and present life events and experiences — in "chain reactions" or continuous stimuli-responses from infancy to adulthood (e.g., upbringing, separation, trauma, memory, reactivation); one thing leads to another in biopsychosocial changes

e) Downloading from culture, education, social media, lifestyle, politics, policy, values, concepts of democracy, human rights, freedom of speech, truths, fakes, etc.

Thus, everything in life is relevant to mental health and psychiatry. Much depends on proper assessment and balance.

Proper psychiatric assessment is **longitudinal** from conception to consultation and includes predisposing, precipitating, perpetuating, and protecting/protective factors. The most appropriate diagnosis is then chosen to fit the patient.

In a forensic issue, the focus is on the individual's mental state at a material point in time or **cross section** assessment, and the "patient" is often made to fit a diagnosis.

As a **clinician's conceptualisation** of clinical presentation **may differ** in focus and understanding, the **diagnosis** made **may not concur** [e.g., in acute stress reaction or disorder (when emphasis is on aetiological stressor), in adjustment disorder (when emphasis is on "change" that is stressful/threatening over time), then cluster of symptomatology, personality pattern/problem, hierarchy of dominant syndrome].

Categories of Mental Disorders have been changing, expanded, controversial, and in a flux. For both DSM-5 and ICD-11, new separate categories/entities are set up or under major disorders and related disorders, such as anxiety or fear related disorders, obsessive-compulsive or related disorders, and impulse control disorders. On the other hand, clinically, some "old" entities are grouped dimensionally into spectrum disorders, such as Asperger's under Autism Spectrum Disorder (ASD). Schizophrenia, schizoaffective disorder, and bipolar disorder have been regarded as a continuum spectrum. In DSM-5, prolonged grief disorder is added as bereavement exclusion from major depression. There are also medicalised inclusions of premenstrual dysphoric disorder, disruptive mood dysregulation disorder, illness anxiety, hoarding, binge eating, and minor neurocognitive disorder.

The principles underlying **ICD** are that it should be clinically useful, global in application, scientifically valid targeting mental health professionals, focused on public health, and ultimately aimed at reducing disease burden worldwide. In the ICD-11, attempts have been made to integrate disorders with onset in childhood and adolescence that continue into adulthood with the main classifications (e.g., ASD, ADHD, psychoses, personality disorders). Efforts have also been made to reduce the number of categories and simplify where possible (e.g., schizophrenic disorders, personality disorder with specifiers). (R. Uher, Canada)

Historically, there have been similar clinical syndromes that were given different names by different people in different cultures and during different periods of time. For instance, the French term "bouffee delirante", the Scandinavian term "psychogenic psychosis", the Anglo-American term "schizoaffective illness", Leonhard's term "cycloid psychosis", and Mitsuda's "atypical psychoses" could all refer to the same group of patients. The term "schizoaffective psychosis" (likewise schizophreniform psychosis, schizotypal disorder, and dysthymia) has also undergone changes in usage over time or apply to different conditions. There is also a hierarchical approach in which a dominant disorder is diagnosed over the presence of concomitant symptoms from another disorder. A more recent trend is to consider the idea of comorbidity or dimensional position occupied. There is also a change in nomenclatures of earlier diagnoses, such as somatoform to somatic or bodily symptoms/disorders and hypochondriasis to illness anxiety.

There has been an increase in the diagnosis of comorbidity due to **cross section** examination of mental state. However, psychopathology should be assessed and understood **developmentally**, **sequentially**, **chronologically**, and **dynamically** to determine what is **primary** and what is **secondary**. This will make management more rational.

Not all mental disorders or conditions are defined and diagnosable by ICD or DSM, hence the category of "not otherwise specified" (NOS) or now "**unspecified**". In clinical practice, variations in diagnostic labels are accepted insofar as the operational criteria are spelt out. However, in research and evaluation, confusion and controversy arise when diagnostic criteria vary or differ. This is because the clinician's conceptualisation of the clinical presentation may differ. Hence, the DSM which provides criteria sets dominates research work. It is also important to be clear about what is a **nosological entity**, a **clinical syndrome**, and a **consensus of opinion**. The implications are far reaching in clinical management, research studies, forensic practice, and insurance coverage or subvention. Both ICD and DSM offer no theoretical discussions or explanations of the causes and effects of classified mental disorders, except perhaps the Disorders specifically associated with stress in the ICD-11.

The human person is so complex that one should avoid forcing square pegs into round holes. The fact that there are many **different** rating scales or measuring instruments and diagnostic inventories or schedules used indicates that no one has exclusive answers. It is often better to be descriptive of the condition and allow room and time for further observation and research. There can be **universal truth** derived from the **studies** of **single cases**. On the other hand, what is **statistically correct** and **significant** may have **no predictive value** for **specific** individuals.

For further reading, refer to Chapter One of *Essential Guide to Psychiatry* on "**Nature of Classification Systems for Psychiatric Disorders**", 2014 by **Dr. Chua Hong Choon**.

2 Mental Functions and Psychopathology

Just as the body (soma) is divided into systems (e.g., central nervous system, cardiovascular system, endocrine system), the mind (psyche) is divided into mental functions, namely **cognitive function, emotion, volition** or **drive,** and **behavioural expression.** These functions are normally **inter-related, interactive, integrated,** and manifested as the individual's psychic experience and physical behaviour. It should be emphasised that the division of body and mind is artificial and undesirable.

Similarly, like the nervous system, which has a hierarchy of organisation and function from the peripheral, spinal, brainstem, sub-cortical to cortical structure, there is also a **hierarchy of development and maturation** of mental life from instinctual, primitive, logical, and rational to intellectual manifestations. Impairment of higher regulatory mechanisms will release an innate response from the lower level systems. This results in what is known as **vegetative function** (neurologically) or **regressive behaviour** (psychologically).

To understand **psychopathology**, which is about **abnormal mental functions**, it is necessary to know what is considered normal (mental) functioning. To begin with, there is cognitive function, which essentially consists of perception, memory, and thinking.

To see an object, there must first be the object, which is the stimulus. Next, there must be adequate lighting, a healthy sensory organ viz. the eye, and an intact neurological pathway for sensation received to reach the unimpaired visual cortex. The stimulus, when completely new, is stored as memory for future reference. If the stimulus is familiar, then it evokes past memory and recognition. This is perception based on past experience. Thinking takes place when ideas associated with the perception are stimulated.

Perception, memory, or thinking may be accompanied by feelings or emotional states that may be pleasant or unpleasant. These **psychological experiences** may elicit **physiological responses** and lead to certain **physical expressions** and **actions** as seen in outward behaviour.

Morbidity can occur anywhere between the stimulus and the behavioural response. The cause of the disorder may be physical and/or psychosocial. The signs and symptoms of psychiatric disorders may be classified according to the mental functions that are disordered. As disorder in one function can affect other functions, secondary symptoms are produced. What one perceives may influence how one feels, which may then determine what one thinks and vice versa. Thus, hallucinatory voices that threaten can lead to fear and secondary delusions of persecution, or feelings of depression can trigger negative thoughts, and so on. Diagnosis is based on the primary disorder or symptoms. However, comorbidity is considered when other coexistent symptoms are also prominent and sustained.

Scheme of Mental Functions

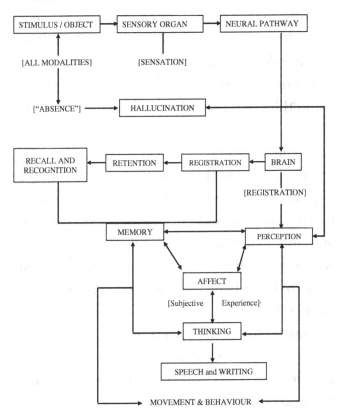

IN CONSCIOUSNESS: (AWARENESS, ATTENTION, CONCENTRATION)

STIMULUS / OBJECT → SENSORY ORGAN → NEURAL PATHWAY

[ALL MODALITIES]   [SENSATION]

["ABSENCE"] → HALLUCINATION

RECALL AND RECOGNITION ← RETENTION ← REGISTRATION ← BRAIN

[REGISTRATION]

MEMORY ← → PERCEPTION

AFFECT

[Subjective   Experience]

THINKING

SPEECH and WRITING

MOVEMENT & BEHAVIOUR

[These normal mental functions are inter-related, interactive, and integrated.]

Disorders of Perception

What is perceived depends on what is there to perceive, environmental factors, and the individual's perceptual habits, mindset, and mental state. Different authors classify and explain psychopathology in slightly different ways. Terms such as distortion, falsification, misinterpretation, and misperception are confusing because of variation in focus and definition. As mentioned earlier, the **integrative** nature of mental functions makes it difficult to distinguish or separate what is perceptual or sensory, what is thinking or ideational, and what is affective or cognitive. Perhaps that is why the same verb **"feel"** (or **"jue 觉"** in mandarin) refers to **sensation/perception** when used "to feel pain or cold"; **emotion/affect** when used "to feel sad or nervous"; and **reasoning/thinking (cognitive)** when used "to feel that it is right or good".

Perception is thus more than sensation as it is closely associated with memory, which incorporates both cognitive and affective aspects of knowing and understanding. Therefore, it is important to accurately observe any phenomenon with an open mind and note its **development, progress**, and the consequent **effect**. What matters essentially is whether the experience or complaint is morbid or non-morbid. Morbidity indicates psychopathology or the result of a disorder in the individual. It can be said that abnormal perceptions arising from a **non-morbid** state (such as due to poor lighting or vision) are considered non-morbid, whereas those arising from a **morbid** state (such as a disordered mind, whether organic or psychological) would be morbid.

Illusions

Under certain circumstances, normal people can experience illusions. An illusion consists of an **object/stimulus** that is **falsely** perceived due to either the lack of clarity of the object/stimulus or the psychological state of the person. Thus, an innocuous silhouette or sound may be perceived as something threatening by someone in a suggestible condition. When the psychological state is morbid, then what is perceived may be misinterpreted, such as in idea of reference. The misperception is understandable and secondary to an underlying morbid state.

The perception of the object/stimulus may be distorted in reality, dimension, or intensity as a result of physical disease or psychiatric disorder. The object/stimulus may appear amplified.

[e.g., hyper-aesthesia (in emotional or physical state)], diminished [e.g., micropsia (in temporal lobe epilepsy)], or strange [e.g., déjà vu (in familiarity)].

Hallucinations

Hallucinations are false "perceptions" in whatever modalities (visual, auditory, olfactory, gustatory, and tactile) where stimuli/objects are **absent** or **non-existent**. The **contents** are important and should be noted. There are many varieties of hallucinations indicative of different organic and mental disorders. Partial seizures are well known to manifest different hallucinatory experiences. **Temporal lobe hallucinations** are multi-sensory but do not include somatic sensations. The primary auditory field lies in this lobe as do parts of the cortical fields for smell and taste. Certain **auditory** hallucinations (e.g., Schneider's first-rank symptoms where patients discuss themselves in the third person, hear their own thoughts being broadcasted, and provide a running commentary on their actions) are diagnostic (but not pathognomonic) of schizophrenia. **Visual** hallucinations are more common in acute **organic** states with clouding of consciousness or **deliriousness** states than in so called "functional" psychoses. They also appear in dementia. Critical or condemning voices may be heard in depressed patients.

Not all hallucinations are morbid in nature (e.g., hypnogogic when falling to sleep, hypnopompic on waking up, and during sensory deprivation). "True" auditory and visual hallucinations are defined as deriving from or occupying real external space. But in **schizophrenia**, patients complain of "voices" coming from certain parts of their bodies (e.g., head, brain, throat, heart). Or they may say that someone is speaking to them through their mouth. Some patients may complain of hearing voices at the beginning of their illness, but these voices disappear later on. When they persist, patients may remark that it is like talking to themselves and not real, and hence they learn to accept and ignore them. **Pseudo-hallucinations** are thought to be more of mental images in internal subjective space and lacking substance. Stated more simply, the patient is aware of the non-reality of these illusions.

Delusional perception starts with normal perception but with **concomitant** formation of **new abnormal ideas** (apophanous) of a delusional nature. For instance, a patient may see someone washing a car and instantaneously believe that gangsters are after him. Such episodes are sometimes preceded by **delusional mood** (feeling of something going on which concerns him). Together with the sudden development or intrusion of a **delusional idea** (out of the blue or **autochthonous**), they form a **primary delusional experience** characteristic of schizophrenia. Delusional perception is therefore not quite the same as misinterpretation of a normal perception as a result of an existing morbid mental state (see also delusional memory below). More often than not, delusional ideas develop or build up, secondary to primary delusional experience, hallucination or mood state, an organic lesion or life situation.

Both hallucination and delusion may be associated with **"unconscious" obsessive rumination** postulated under Obsessive-Compulsive Disorder.

Disorders of Memory

The formation of normal memory begins with attention to and normal perception of a stimulus or subject material. Then there has to be proper registration, consolidation, and retention of the perception and material for future recall when required. Any stage of the memory formation process may be affected for various reasons, such as poor attention and concentration, mood state, brain diseases, drugs, emotional conflict, and normal forgetting. In addition, the left brain is more concerned with verbal memory and the right brain with visual-spatial memory. During learning or acquisition of new knowledge and skill, memory would necessarily undergo revision or edition.

Impairment of memory in general indicates **organic** disorders including delirium, dementia, brain disease, head injury, and effect of drugs/alcohol. However, memory function can also be disturbed when normal processes of **registration, retention,** and **retrieval** (or encoding, consolidation, and retrieval) are affected by particular mental states. In situations of distraction, deficits of attention and concentration, and emotional conflicts such as anxiety, depression, and dissociative disorders, memory disturbances are frequently complained of with fear of brain damage or disease. Depending on the cause, amnesia may be **anterograde, retrograde, subjective, reversible,** or **permanent**. Like the computer, a file may be "lost" because of faulty saving or corruption but subsequently retrieved through different pathways.

Memory can also be falsified in that what is remembered had in fact never happened or is not exactly as it was. **Deja vu**, in which there is a sense of familiarity in a new place, would be one such example. In **confabulation**, fabricated or false answers are given to questions regarding the past because of amnesia. **Delusional**

memory is the development of a delusion alongside normal memory. It is similar in concept to delusional perception of the primary delusional experience. (The concept may possibly be extended to that of a "**delusional dream**".)

Memory is generally considered part of cognition, but due to the associations between mental functions (see Memory and Reflex), there are also **affective, sensory,** and **motor** memories. Thus, past emotional experiences can be provoked and relived when particular events are recalled. On the other hand, the affective component of the experience may be separated and repressed, or appear in a different guise that is **dissociated** from the **"cognitive"** memory.

Disorders of Thinking

Thinking involves association of ideas and is expressed in **speech** or **writing** for communication. However, in order to respond and communicate, the capacity to understand what is heard or read must be intact. In a psychiatric setting, disorders of thinking cause breakdowns in communication that are unrelated to coarse organic lesions, intellectual functioning, language ability or barrier, or cultural difference.

Frank Fish classifies disorders of thinking according to:

1. **Stream/Flow** — whether **rapid** or **slow**, and its **direction/ goal** (e.g., flight of ideas with chance associations in mania; retardation of speech in depression)
2. **Possession/Ownership** — **involuntary** or **alien** in nature (e.g., obsessional ruminations or thought insertion/withdrawal/ broadcast as in Schizophrenia, respectively)
3. **Content** — what is expressed (i.e., **delusional** ideas that may be persecutory, grandiose, nihilistic, erotic, or of jealousy) that

is systematised or illogical as in regressive primary thinking, such as active dreaming

4. **Form** — how words and ideas are associated or linked

Formal Thought Disorders

These refer particularly to those found in schizophrenia, though they can also occur in coarse brain disease. The central feature is **disconnection**. If thought is "words forming ideas", then examples ranging from the worst to the subtlest type of thought disorder are as follows:

Neologism — letters of the alphabet put together but not forming words (or ordinary words used differently/peculiarly)

Word salad — words thrown together but not forming sentences

Disjointed talk — no logical connection between sentences

Dissociation of ideas — paragraphs loosely linked or out of context

Vagueness in speech — talk or answers that are seemingly logical or relevant but are difficult to follow and lead nowhere

Studies indicate that formal thought disorder can also occur in normal people.

In "**perplexity**", the patient appears unable to register and understand what is said to him or make the necessary response. It is like a computer system that has hanged, a page of printed words gone out of alignment, or sentences broken up. Sometimes, the patient may respond with "Huh?" or may answer the first few words clearly but later fizzle out in mumbles like a radio with weak batteries. Or there may be cross-reception and interference due to poor differentiation of channel frequencies.

In **circumstantiality**, the person does not come to the point directly. There is much beating around the bush and giving of a lot of details before finally answering the question. When the answer goes off the point completely, it becomes **tangential**.

Disorders of Moods

What or how one feels or reacts depends on individual predispositions, which are a part of personality traits and external factors in the environment. There is a range of emotional experiences and behaviour in sadness, joy, anger, and fear that is considered appropriate and normal.

However, when the moods of **depression** (low spirit), **elation** (high spirit), or **irritability** are out of proportion in intensity and duration, dominate or overwhelm the individual, and affect his normal functioning, then a mood disorder exists. **Primary mood disorder** has **secondary effects** on other important functions such as thinking, memory, and behaviour. Sometimes a mood disorder is not apparent unless the "**emotional baseline**" of the individual is known (e.g., extroverted or introverted). It could also be an **acute on chronic situation**; that is, the so called "**double depression**".

In psychotic conditions, mood may be **incongruous**. Patients may laugh or cry without appropriate reasons and feelings or complain that when they see/hear happy things, they cry and conversely when they see/hear sad things, they laugh. **Affective blunting**, which is characteristic if not diagnostic of schizophrenia, shows a **lack of sensitivity** in feeling and has a quality of indifference or callousness to it. **Flattening of affect** is a **loss of expressivity** of feeling, such as masked facies in Parkinsonism, and which can be induced by neuroleptics. However, some may use blunting and flattening interchangeably. "**La belle indifference**" is typically described in conversion disorders in which the patient shows an inappropriate lack of concern about his disability.

Disorders of Consciousness

Consciousness is the **awareness** of self and the environment. When the awareness is focused, it is **attention** (like the pointing cursor) and when the attention is sustained, it is **concentration.** Normally, when an individual is in control of his mind, he is able to shift his attention at will to concentrate on any immediate task at hand. Other objects or intrusions are kept out. In other words, at any point of time, there would be a dominant consciousness and possibly a hierarchy of subsidiary consciousness in the background. This "subconscious" mind (like programmed functions and applications in the computer, running in the background and out of sight) may distract or intrude from time to time (like advertisements, messages, or prompting) into the conscious mind or monitor screen.

The mind works like a multi-tasking computer with windows being opened, minimised, or toggled according to applications or requirements. Consciousness may also be split as when one sings a song and thinks of something else at the same time. However, when the mind is disturbed or over-aroused, for instance by life events, highly expressed emotions, excessive stimuli, and other activities, it loses control over what the dominant consciousness should be. Other covert mental processes become overt and manifest independently as various forms of psychopathology. Again, it is like a computer with too many windows opened in succession and the CPU processing slows down, hangs, or crashes. These "independent" mental processes may dominate, interfere, or co-exist with the "normal" mind and blur its boundaries. Some patients can recognise these abnormal mental processes and learn to overcome them by avoiding or taking breaks from excessive input.

Under **physiological** conditions, the lowering of consciousness (e.g., dimming of light) leads to **sleep. Clouding of consciousness** is **pathological** as awareness, attention, and concentration (i.e., mental clarity) are affected and may result in a **comatose** state. **Confusion** is clouding of consciousness with **disorientation**. It is obvious that other mental functions (i.e., perception, thinking, feeling) are also affected. Hallucinations are present, thinking is disordered, and the patient exhibits fear and restlessness as in **delirium**.

There is **variation** in different textbooks and past literatures by various authors on the **concept** and **definition** of "confusion" and "delirium". The two words have different historical streams and backgrounds. From historical Continental **(French)** psychiatry, the term "confusion" has a wide meaning, and it likely includes the **British** description of "delirium" as it is commonly understood and used.

The term "**confusion**" may have a number of connotations. In the **ordinary sense**, it means a **lack of comprehension** or simply "I do not understand". The possible reasons for confusion include low intellectual capacity, linguistic difficulty, lack of information, unfamiliarity with the subject matter, or poor communication between parties. The instructed/listening person who complains shows insight and the communicator may lack awareness of his shortcomings in clarity, grasp, and skill in delivery.

Clinical terms of "**confusion**" may also be applied descriptively to patients with mental disorders, and the hallmarks of confusion are **chaotic thinking** and **cognitive failure**. For example, in schizophrenia, confusion is more likely to be due to perplexity, thought disorder, and hallucinatory distraction. In retarded depression, it may be related to the restriction of attention and poor concentration, and in mania it may be a result of hyperactive distractions. There may also be interference from agitated and amnesic states. The use of the word confusion **does not, by itself** indicate the presence or absence of altered consciousness.

The clinical term "**delirium**", however, is understood definitively as a psychopathology of consciousness. It regards the presence of "**clouding of consciousness**" as the essential core of pathophysiology (incidentally, a pivotal paper by Chaslin and Bonhoeffer brought the two concepts of confusion and delirium together as features of **acute brain failure**). Delirium is like groping around in poor lighting and trying to operate electronic gadgets when the battery is running low. The aetiology or pathogenesis is **organic** in basis. The medical or physical conditions include infection, inflammation, trauma, substance intoxication/withdrawal, organ failure, metabolic disorders, coarse brain disease, post-general anaesthesia, ECT, etc., resulting in loss of independent/voluntary control and brain function.

In confusion and delirium, brain processes are disordered and cognitive function is impaired. In our practice, the operational clinical test for confusion is disorientation in person, place, and time. Clarity of thought, perception, and memory are affected.

In delirium due to impairment of cognitive functions, there is pathology of consciousness, perceptual disturbance, and distortion resulting in hallucination, illusion, and delusional ideas such as threat. There may be affective responses associated with "fear, frenzy, and freezing" and psychomotor/behavioural reactions. One's individual personality make-up and past experience may influence the manifestation. The delirious state fluctuates and reacts to external cues in the environment, such as lighting, movement, and sound. Hence, a calm and well-lit environment and measured intervention are helpful in management.

A digital camera with weak battery power would be erratic and inaccurate in computing data. Pictures taken would turn out underexposed and unfocused. Likewise in confusion and delirium, because of clouding of consciousness, there would be blurred or even absent memory.

Consciousness may also be **restricted** as in a dissociative or fugue state, which can be unconsciously caused or when under hypnosis.

In **self-consciousness**, there is awareness and insight of one's appearance, feeling, thinking, speech, and behaviour in relation to the environment and others. Self-consciousness or **non-self-consciousness** may be normal or abnormal depending on the mental state of the individual. There may be variable sensitivity toward or delusional interpretations about others and the environment, or indifference and oblivion in psychotic behaviour.

Other Disturbances of Self Awareness

Depersonalisation

Depersonalisation is a feeling or sense of **change** in oneself, whether **emotionally** or **physically**, with an **unpleasant** quality. It also includes **derealisation**, which refers to the same phenomenon but of the environment. This sense of **dissonant** change in oneself or the environment may be due to the **dissociation** between **cognition** and **affect** and **dissociation of affect** with **loss of feeling**. For instance, one patient may say, "I know it is raining outside but I am unable to feel that it is so." Another says, "I am worried because I should be feeling sad, but I am not." Yet another who is panting away after exercise says, "I am unable to feel breathless."

On the other hand, although patients are unable to **subjectively** feel emotions, their **external emotional expressions** or

responses appear to be quite **normal.** Thus, they may laugh heartily at a joke and yet state that they cannot perceive the humour. In normal functioning, we think, feel, and behave in **consonance.**

Identity and Boundary

These are psychotic phenomena in which the patient thinks he is someone other than himself, his body is not his own, he has no control over his thoughts and feelings, or there is mutual influence of action and behaviour between himself and the environment. For instance, an engineer may empathise strongly with an overworked train, or another patient may complain that movement observed around her makes her feel uncomfortable/unwell in the left half of her head and body.

Passivity Experience

Schizophrenia sufferers may complain of being **made** to think, feel, and act in certain ways by some external force outside voluntary control. It has to be differentiated from compulsive behaviour and disorder of thinking and mood. One abnormal offender explained that he was made to throw a child down the building.

Motor Disorders

Generally, our actions and responses are intentional, purposeful, and adaptive. However, in some coarse brain diseases and mental disorders, the individual's posture, movement, behaviour, facial expression, and speech or utterance may become disordered because of **neurological lesion** or **psychological "blocking/obstruction"** in their spontaneous and smooth execution. **Catatonic symptoms** from hyperkinesis to akinesis and from abnormal posture to behaviour and response are outward physical signs that may have neurological as well as psychopathological basis. As such, they are also termed "**psychomotor disorder**". The "flow" of movement and response may become interrupted or repetitive as in perseveration. **Mannerism** is used to describe seemingly goal-oriented behaviour and may reflect personal characteristics. **Stereotypy** refers to apparently non-adaptive or non-goal-oriented behaviour or movement.

However, because mannerism may merge into stereotypy, it is not always easy to distinguish the two. In speech, echolalia (echoing what is said), palilalia (repeating the last word), logoclonia (repeating the last syllable of the last word), and echopraxia (copying actions) are classic examples. In **stupor**, the patient is mute, motionless, and unresponsive to stimulation to varying degrees. The differential causes are organic, psychotic or catatonic, psychogenic or hysterical, and affective (manic or depressive). **Catatonia** is a differential diagnosis of stupor that is most commonly seen in catatonic schizophrenia. The clinical picture may range from "frozen" to "frenzied" or excitable. The presence of incontinence of urine and faeces would be indicative of organic or psychotic conditions. **Cataplexy** may be considered a "perseveration of posture" induced in catatonia.

A Neuropsychological Model

Neuronal (or Neural) Circuits and Networks

There are probably up to 100 billion neurons with up to 100 trillion synapses estimated in the human brain. In addition, about 100 neurotransmitters have been discovered. Each neuron is connected to many other neurons, forming myriads of neural circuits and networks. There is continuous attrition of nerve cells and there may also be birth of new ones through neurogenesis.

The brain receives nerve impulses continuously from both external and internal environments through the sense organs of the body. Every stimulus of adequate threshold must necessarily be transmitted through chains of neurons. The impulses of different modalities converge in a **network of neuronal circuits**, which integrate them into meaningful information and evoke appropriate responses through familiar or newly created neuronal circuits. Like well-trodden footpaths, the circuitry may become **stereotyped** or go into **default**.

Neuronal (neural) connections are mediated through **neurotransmitters**, which may lead to **excitatory** or **inhibitory** impulses in different parts of the complex network of neuronal circuits to induce appropriate stimuli and responses. However, for various reasons including metabolic disturbance, inflammatory processes, and the dying of brain cells, there may be **excessive** or **deficient** excitation or inhibition that results in disruption and malfunction. One simplified explanation is based on the availability and balance of neurotransmitters and receptors. In Parkinsonism, there is a deficiency of dopamine in the basal ganglia and an imbalance of dopamine and acetylcholine. In depressive illness, it is believed that there is deficiency of biogenic amines at the synaptic junctions, and in schizophrenia, there is dopaminergic overactivity in the mesolimbic system or hypoactivity in the mesocortical pathway. In the dementing process, the loss of neurons results in permanent break up of circuitry and destruction of mental function.

Memory and Reflex

Memory is a cognitive function. It involves registration (encoding) of stimulus (whether external or internal), which is received by sense organs (of whatever modality) and conveyed through nerves to some specific area(s) in the brain. By some complex processes, the information or psychic experience is stored or retained (as synaptic and systemic consolidation) for future recall. A memory trace is thus formed, so to speak.

When we read silently for instance, the visual pathway is activated. If we read aloud, then the auditory pathway as well as the sensorimotor pathway of the articulatory apparatus is opened up. In addition, if we write or copy the words that are being vocalised and the passage evokes certain emotional responses, then more neurological pathways are called into play. The whole neurophysiological process is further influenced by circumstances that surround the individual. There may be other competing, distracting, or soothing audio-visual, tactile, thermal, olfactory, autonomic, and psychic stimuli (e.g., music, lighting, temperature setting, aroma, health state, or influence of a significant person). Each stimulus could possibly generate specific nerve impulses that travel in specific pathways, forming a circuit and its own memory trace. All these circuits may **antagonise, interfere, reinforce,** or **integrate** with one another. The "**final memory**" is the "**convergent product**" of all these inputs.

The **complete** or **partial recall** of this "convergent" memory may be triggered by one or more of the **component sensory stimuli** that are associated like a **set piece**, such as the total experience of a memorable candlelight dinner, musical extravaganza, or beautiful holiday. Thus, during communication, there is not only vocal speech but also emotional expression, body language, and gesticulation even when talking to someone on the telephone. On the other hand, one or more of these component circuits may go into "loops", get shunted, short circuit, become entangled or disconnected, or for one reason or another (medical or psychological) exist separately and function independently. The result can cause the various "**split**" and **incongruous phenomena** and **repetitive symptoms** that are seen in depersonalisation syndrome, schizophrenia, obsessive-compulsive disorder, or addictive behaviour. Instead of being "convergent", the memory is now "**divergent**". Subsequently, when the "**trace**" is set, the memory becomes a "**reflex**". However, memory is not static or permanent; it can undergo modification and edition with new experiences, developments, and applications.

A reflex is a fixed **stimulus-response** that may be conditioned or learned. A typical reflex action (e.g., knee jerk) is said to be at the "spinal" level and does not involve consciousness. However, this is not completely true. Many patterns of behaviour, habits, responses, and skills, such as driving, games and sports, and musical scales and scores, are first consciously and deliberately learned and practised before they become automatic. Correction is difficult later on when the "memory trace" is too entrenched. On the other hand, **a conscious thought** or **an unconscious desire** may initiate an **outflow of neurological impulses** that can be recorded or observed in the behavioural response of the target organs. This can be a principle for robotic prosthesis.

Cognitive Functions and Photography

The brain is like the film and memory is like the picture taken. The level of consciousness is like the degree of brightness or intensity of light. When lighting is poor or absent, the picture will be blurred or blank. Hence, at different levels of consciousness, there will be varying degrees of subsequent amnesia. To get good pictures, the lens must be clear and the focusing and exposure must be correct. Similarly, memory function depends on intact sensory organs and neurological pathways as well as directed attention and concentration. When freshly exposed film is developed straight away, the pictures will be vivid. Similarly, when learning is quickly rehearsed, the memory becomes better consolidated, but if the film is double exposed or the developing is much delayed, then the pictures are superimposed or faded. In the same way, if learning is distracted and interfered with or what has been learned is left unused, then the memory is muddled or lost. When the brain is aged and damaged as in dementia, it is like a roll of film that has expired; therefore, the memory or image is impaired. Finally, perception and memory are influenced by the mood state just like the tone of the picture is coloured by the filter.

Fundamental Theories of Psychoanalysis

Psychoanalysis is:

1. A technique of **free association** used in psychotherapy — the patient is encouraged to speak his mind or say whatever thought that comes into his consciousness without censorship.
2. A theory constructed by Freud to explain the materials that emerged in psychotherapy — it becomes, in some sense, a **Personality Theory**.

Sigmund Freud (1856–1939) had early training and research in neuroanatomy, neuropathology, neurology, and hypnosis. His theories are physical in basis and approach.

Basic Assumptions or Hypotheses

1. **Psychic determinism or causality**
   Each psychic event is determined by events that preceded it, just as all physical events have causal determinants. It is therefore important to trace the origin or primary cause.
2. **Theory of the Unconscious**
   Mind
   (a) Conscious: like the tip of a visible iceberg or the visible running applications of a computer
   (b) Unconscious: instinctual forces and repressed conflicts, like the hidden, submerged bulk of an iceberg or what is in the hard disk of a computer

3. **Mechanism of Repression**
Unconscious suppression of what is painful or threatening to one's wellbeing, image, or self-esteem. Successful repression leads to neurotic symptoms while failure to repress results in psychotic breakdown.

Structure of the Personality (Mind)

1. **Id — Original System of Personality**
Reservoir of all psychic energy (like the CPU)

Mode of operation:
Pleasure Principle — immediate gratification of instinctual needs and reduction of psychic tension regardless of the realistic situation
Primary Process Thinking (or communication) — direct, immediate, disinhibited, uncensored, non-verbal, and reality-fantasy (blurring or mixing); beyond logic, objectivity, contradiction, space, and time. (pictorial, imagery)
"**I WANT (NOW)!**" e.g., something direct from the TV screen.

2. **EGO — Executive Part of Personality**
Derives from the Id and is mostly conscious. It is the Mediator between the Id, the Outside World (or reality), the Superego, past memories, and the body's physical needs.

Mode of operation:
Reality Principle — to test or assess reality, evaluate and plan, and modify or censor accordingly
Secondary Process Thinking (or communication) — may be indirect, delayed, and matured in meeting the demand/desired goal; verbal, logical, and objective.
"**CAN I HAVE?**" ("Let me see".)

3. SUPEREGO — Moral Part of Personality

Post Oedipal, partly conscious, and consists of:

a. Conscience → guilt feeling
b. Ego-ideal → deep inner feelings of wellbeing and pride. It incorporates
   (1) basic moral principles and ideals of parents, and
   (2) basic values or traditions of cultures.

"SHOULD I HAVE?" ("Is it good/right?").

Topography of Personality (Mind)

1. **Conscious** — Parts of mental life or experience that the individual is readily aware of at any given moment. It includes most but not all of the Ego (cf., open applications on the computer).
2. **Preconscious** — Parts of mental life that can be brought into consciousness with concentration and effort. It lies principally in the Ego (cf., minimised applications on the computer).
3. **Unconscious** — Parts of mental life that are totally outside awareness. Contents may remain permanently unknown, or parts of it may at times pass into the preconscious and from there be called up into the conscious. Contents are primarily behaviour and thought determined by the Id and the Superego. The unconscious Ego produces the mechanism of defense and symptoms formation. Evidence of unconscious mind derives from slip of the tongue, dreams, free association, narcoanalysis, hypnosis, and psychotic symptoms.

Dynamics of Personality

Psychic Energy is the subjective experience of power and enthusiasm, and is the hypothetical driving force responsible for all psychological actions.

Instinct (Freud)

At first: only **Sex instinct** → source of all instinctual drives

Later: propounded **Two instincts** —

1. Eros — group of self-preservation drives (mainly sexual)
2. Thanatos — self-destructive, aggressive group of drives

Most of Freud's followers:

1. Aggressive drives cannot be entirely derived from sexual instinct
2. Reject self-destructive (or death) instinct — Thanatos

> Thus **Id = Instincts + Psychic Energy**. (Ego and Superego also derive from the Id and depend on its energy source)

A. **Instincts:** All stem from the Id
1. **Sexual instinct** ("Libido", "Life instinct" — Eros) is the drive for: Individual gratification and racial propagation

Pleasurable and creative activities

Has a somatic basis in the **erogenous zones** of the body. The energy associated with the sexual instinct is the **libido**, which forms a **major part** of psychic energy. It is a **psycho-physiological** process with both **mental** and **physical** manifestations.

Libido — refers to the force by which the sexual instinct is represented in the mind (i.e., mental manifestation of sexual instinct).

2. **Aggressive instinct**. Includes all the hostile and destructive forces in the human psyche. Derivatives include the impulse to self-assertion, ambition, competition, the desire to win, and the drive to succeed. Sexual and aggressive drives may fuse.

Energy Concepts — Psychic energy distributed among the Id, the Ego, and the Superego in different ways in different individuals.

Cathexis — Psychic energy directed to or invested in an object (person or thing) or function (e.g., one's work with the purpose of gratifying an instinct or its derivative)

B. Anxiety

1. **Realistic** Anxiety — fear of real dangers in the external world
2. **Neurotic** Anxiety — fear of instincts getting out of control (e.g., aggression) and leading to punishment
3. **Moralistic** Anxiety — fear of conscience resulting in guilt.

Free Floating Anxiety

"**Neurotic**" **functions** to prevent the conscious part of the Ego from recognising actual specific conflict situations in a pathological attempt to "protect" the Ego from the conflict.

Traumatic Anxiety

When the Ego becomes overwhelmed and ineffective → defense mechanism — which may be normal or abnormal (e.g., rationalisation or regression; see "defense mechanism" on page **25**)

Signal Anxiety

Early preconscious perception of anxiety by the Ego that leads to the initiation of protective measures to prevent the development of a full-blown anxiety state.

Therefore, it would not be inappropriate to say that Anxiety is the "Mother of Psychopathology" and is in some way or other involved in most mental disorders.

Bowlby *et al.* (1969, 1973, 1980, 1988) believe that like all mammals, human infants are genetically predisposed to want access or proximity to an **attached figure.** Excessive fear and distress are triggered and experienced due to **separation anxiety.** Being totally dependent on the caregiver in early life, any threat to the child's sense of security will activate the attachment system, resulting in the characteristic sequence of **protest, despair,** and **detachment** behaviour.

Lindermann (1944) first defined psychological trauma as "sudden uncontrollable disruption of our affiliative bonds."

Chronic HPA (hypothalamic-pituitary-adrenal) stress response is toxic.

[Early prevention, diagnosis and treatment (**ASAP**) are therefore important.]

A — Attachment to source of mothering and nurturing to ensure survival and security during infancy and early childhood [Protective]

S — Separation from/**Scarring** of attachment [Predisposing]

A — Activation/Anticipation of separation anxiety by trauma and threat [Precipitating]

P — Psychopathology [conversion/dissociation as in hysteria; avoidance of object and situation as in phobias; ritual/undoing as in OCD in defense; GAD in failure to contain anxiety]

Development of the Personality in response to three major sources of tension:

A. **Physiological growth processes** (including infantile sexuality — "Oedipal Complex" and resolution)

B. **External frustrations of drives**

C. **Internal conflicts between dynamic forces**

THEORY OF PERSONALITY

Topography / Structure	Unconscious (e.g., hard disk)	Pre-conscious (e.g., minimised applications)	Conscious (e.g., opened applications)	External
Id (original system: instincts and psychic energy)	Pleasure principle: (immediate gratification) Primary thinking process			
Ego (Regulates between internal needs and external reality) **CPU (Brain)**	Defense — mechanisms Symptoms formation → ←	→ ←	Reality principle: Evaluate/ Execute Mediate/ Co-ordinate Endorse/ Censor Secondary thinking process	Outside World Reality
Superego (Post Oedipal)	Conscience/ ego-ideal (introjection)		Moral standards Values/ Ideals	
	(Nonverbal and repression)		(Verbal)	

Psychosexual Development

Infantile Sexuality

"Sexual" includes all kinds of pleasures that the child obtains from his bodily sensations. Activities at different stages of development are focused on different muco-cutaneous junction areas of the body and are known as oral, anal, and phallic stages of libidinal development. The infant desires gratification of the instinctual needs connected with a given stage (but it may not have the same connotation of adult sexuality).

Pre-Oedipal Phase (birth to about age 4):
1. **Oral Phase** (birth to age 1–2 years).
Primary interest centred on **mouth** (e.g., sucking, biting, mouthing, swallowing, eating, chewing, drinking, talking, kissing, spitting, smoking, etc.)

Infant — **narcissistic** (only aware of and concerned with the self)
Pleasures — **autoerotic** (stimulation of self)
Goals — development of **basic trust** and **security**
Ego boundary (body ego)
Psychopathology — oral aggression ("fed like an infant") distortion, hallucination, denial, projection, etc.

2. **Anal Phase** (age 1–3)
Libidinal energies centred on retention and expulsion of faeces [i.e., control of anal sphincter to please or displease parents (**obedience/defiance**)]; still **narcissistic and autoerotic**.

Goals — **autonomy** and **control** (bowel training); **ego formation**
Psychopathology — as in obsessive-compulsive behaviour, indecision, ambivalence, sado-masochistic behaviour.
Mechanism used — displacement, reaction formation, undoing, and isolation

3. **Phallic Phase** (age 3–5)
Libidinal energies focused on penis and clitoris and concerned with **power** and **strength.** Initially autoerotic but later changes into differentiated sexual interest on the opposite-sex parent. It is the **beginning of the oedipal period.**

Goal — Self-initiation; formation of Superego

Psychopathology — sexual deviancy

4. Urethral Phase (age 3–5)

It coincides with late anal and phallic stages and involves interest and concern with bladder control, leading to the phenomenon of **shame** (i.e., enuresis)

Symbolic — setting fires and putting them out; having aggressive and masturbatory elements

Oedipal Phase (age 3–4 to 6–7)

Development of **sexual interest** in **parent of opposite sex** and consequently strong feelings of rivalry towards parent of same sex. However, forbidden sexual desires and feelings of **love/hate** towards parent of same sex produce feelings of anxiety and guilt and fear of punishment for the "crime". This results in **castration anxiety** and **oedipal conflict.**

   Resolution — repression of sexual feelings; identifying with parts of each parent (i.e., **moral** and **idealistic** values of each parent). This formation of the Superego is largely unconscious.

   Ego of Male child — "I cannot literally have mother for my own but I can make part of her (conscience and ideals) become part of me. Then I will possess her in this safe way. Likewise I cannot do away with father whom I both love and hate but I can become like him (by taking over his conscience and ideals) and then he will like me and no longer see me as a rival and hence will not castrate me. Mother will even like me more since in this non-sexual manner I have become more like father who is her real lover."

   Psychopathology — over-attachment, over-identification, undue fear of parent, poorly resolved oedipal phase → poorly formed or deficient Superego → sociopathic character disorders and neuroses. Psychoses (psychological aspect) generally stem from earlier oedipal problems.

Reasons for poorly resolved oedipal period:

a. Entering oedipal phase with too many **unresolved pre-oedipal conflicts** (oral, anal, phallic) so that not enough psychic energy is available to deal effectively with this new phase.
b. **Absence of either parent** (without a good substitute; i.e., no model).
c. Severe psychopathology in either parent (i.e., **poor or bad model**).

Latency Period — (age 7–12 to 14)
A period of relative sexual quiescence follows resolution of oedipal period. Sexual fantasies and activities are repressed.

> **Genital Phase** (adolescent phase)
> From autoerotic (phallic phase) transformed to **love object** and development of **identity, maturity**, and **independence**.

Fixation and Regression:

Fixation may occur at any phase of development and result in psychic energy being tied down. Difficulties resulting in fixation include over-frustration, over-gratification, and gross inconsistencies (from key figures).

> **Regression** occurs when one retreats to an earlier phase of development (to a point of fixation) when faced with stressful situations.

> **Analogy** It is like building a house with some given amount of materials (i.e., psychic/libidinal energy) and scheduled periods of time (i.e., developmental stages). Different individuals may concentrate on (or neglect) certain areas of the house such

as the kitchen (oral), bathroom/toilet (anal/urethral), bedroom (phallic), or living-room (genital) and apportion different quantities of materials and time to their construction, resulting in an unbalanced house that cannot adequately fulfil its complete purpose. It is to be expected that depending on the care and materials invested, some areas would be well constructed and strong while the other areas would be deficient and weak. When stressed or during crisis, the individual will retreat to his/her favourite part of the house.

Fixation Point refers to a "**weak spot**" left behind by unresolved conflict from under- or over-gratification during a given stage. Conflict is reactivated when experiencing stress in adult life.

Defense Mechanism of the Ego:

REPRESSION is the underlying basis of all of defense mechanisms. It is an **unconscious** process.

Through repression, the Ego keeps threatening impulses, feelings, conflicts, wishes, fantasies, and memories from becoming conscious and troubling the individual.

The other defense mechanisms are essentially various types of Ego activity that assist in maintaining repression.

The **Ego** at all times attempts to cope with **three sources of stress:**

1. **Id** — constant push for instinctual gratification
2. **Superego** — constant reminder of good and bad
3. **Outside reality** — multiple external demands

The Ego attempts to deal with these using the best and most efficient methods at its disposal:

a. Conscious — **logical** and **rational** approach based on learned knowledge and past experiences

b. Utilises various **defense mechanisms** acquired in development and unconsciously brought into play by the Ego (e.g., forgetfulness, excuses, avoidance)

c. Ego utilises **symptom formation** (e.g., anxiety, depression, phobias, obsession), which is a pathological attempt by the Ego to deal with extant problems after other methods have failed.

Transference — **rekindling/reactivation** of past emotional attitudes or responses towards certain **key** figures is directed to someone else (e.g., therapist) because of some specific similarity. Transference is an **unconscious** process and may be **positive** or **negative.**

Counter-transference — when the therapist feels likewise towards the patient.

Roles

From childhood, we have been learning and cultivating roles consciously and unconsciously, voluntarily and involuntarily. We are influenced by what we "download" from society and our experiencess. When we meet and interact with others, it is always at many levels. We play many roles and switch roles constantly to match the situation we are in. It is almost a reflex.

It is not often realised that the relationship between two persons as lovers is not the same as when they are husband and wife. This is again different when they become parents. There are implied obligations and responsibilities in each relationship. Thus, the relationship between the same persons is not constant but changes with assumption of new roles. Perhaps, this is why some people choose marriage to start a family while others prefer cohabitation or even single parenthood to maintain the status quo of certain relationships.

On the other hand, each society has its own concept of the necessity and expectation of roles. In addition, not only do relationships change with changing roles, but each role itself also undergoes change with time, such as the role of a husband or wife, parent or child, or teacher or pupil. It has much implications for duty, parenting, and educating.

Post Freudian

Since Freud, many other psychoanalytical or psychodynamic schools have developed, focusing and elaborating on or modifying different aspects of his hypotheses based on the individual founder's observations, experiences, and beliefs. A consequence is that sometimes the same term (e.g., "introjection") is used differently by different authors.

3 Psychiatric Consultations

Psychiatric consultation ranges from **problems in living** to **neurosis, psychosis**, and **organic brain syndrome**. In fact, in **liaison psychiatry**, it covers virtually the whole of medicine and human activities. Our psychiatric practice is **phenomenological** in approach. **Accurate observation** and **reliable description** of the development and progress of signs and symptoms are therefore of paramount importance. There is no substitute for a complete and detailed longitudinal case history. The **stigma** of mental illness is universal and dies hard. People often seek psychiatric treatment as a last resort. Patients and their relatives and friends alike are therefore inclined to deny the mental afflictions and attribute them to some cultural beliefs or other plausible explanations. We should distinguish **objective facts** from **subjective understanding** or **interpretation**. As a matter of fact, the more factual information or data is available, the less the need to hypothesise or resort to complex bio-statistics. To achieve this, curiosity, diligence, and thoroughness in interviews are essential. The psychiatrist is his own laboratory, subject to his experience, knowledge, and skill. The development and use of rating scales are akin to laboratory tests for more objective assessments. Only then can we come to a proper diagnostic formulation and carry out appropriate treatment. It is believed that knowing the **mechanism** of mental disorder may replace phenomenology.

Referral and Admission

The following is with reference to practice in Singapore.
Patients requiring consultation or admission may be referred to the Institute of Mental Health (IMH)/Woodbridge Hospital (WH), its specialist clinics, and community wellness clinics from any source. Non-emergency cases should preferably be referred by appointment to specialist clinics in IMH/WH or one of the designated community wellness clinics nearer to their homes. Walk-ins without appointments must be prepared to wait for available doctors on duty. Consultation fees are chargeable.

For emergency cases, the Medical Officer on duty will use his discretion and judgement to examine the patients in order of urgency. The police and the ambulance should not be kept waiting too long and the disturbed patients should be attended to early. When **violence** is anticipated, the special squad should be summoned immediately. Meanwhile keep calm, be reassuring, and do not provoke. Sometimes it is necessary to admit the disturbed or violent patient first and examine him later in the ward. Do not hesitate to consult or ask for help from the senior doctors at any time.

Guidelines for Admission

As a rule, admission should be on a voluntary basis. However, the following persons or patients are admitted involuntarily or formally:

A. Warrant of Remand

Those who are sent from the **Court** with a Warrant of Remand are admitted for psychiatric assessment. It is usually for a period of two to three weeks, but can be extended if necessary. Medical reports regarding **soundness of mind** in **criminal responsibility** and **fitness to plead** are expected. Others are admitted under special detention orders. They all go to the **forensic** wards.

However, "**Category A**" patients, whether brought by the police or Singapore Armed Forces, are not to be admitted. They have their own arrangements.

B. *Mental Health (Care and Treatment) ACT (2008)*

This new Act replaces or repeals the Mental Disorders and Treatment Act (1985). It provides for the **detention**, **care**, and **treatment** of mentally disordered persons in **designated** psychiatric institutions. "**Treatment**" includes **observation**, **inpatient treatment**, **outpatient treatment**, and **rehabilitation**.

It is the duty of the **police officer** to apprehend any person who is reported to be **mentally disordered**, believed to be **dangerous** to himself or other persons by reason of mental disorder, and take the person together with a report of the facts of the case to any **designated medical practitioner** at a ("**gazetted**") **psychiatric institution**, after which the designated medical practitioner may act in accordance with **Section 10**.

"**Mental disorder**" refers to any mental illness or any other disorder or disability of the mind, and "mentally disordered" shall be construed accordingly.

"**Psychiatric institution**" refers to a psychiatric institution designated by the Minister under **Section 3**. It may be any hospital or any part of a hospital (including psychiatric outpatient clinics).

The **Magistrate**, when provided with evidence of **cruel treatment** or **neglect** of **mentally disordered person**, may make an **order** for the person to be sent to a designated medical practitioner as above who thereafter may act in accordance with Section 10.

In addition, officially approved letters/memos are available for IMH doctors to request for police help to bring mentally disordered persons/patients to the Emergency Services at the IMH/WH for action under the Mental Health (Care and Treatment) Act Chapter 178A. (This letter is valid for one week from the date of referral.)

In **Section 10**, a designated medical practitioner at a (**gazetted**) psychiatric institution, after examining any person who is suffering from a mental disorder and is of the opinion that he/she **should be treated**, or **continue to be treated**, as an **inpatient** at the psychiatric institution, may at any time sign an order in accordance with **Form 1**. This applies to both **at admission for treatment** as well as **for detention and further treatment of an inpatient**.

Form 1   signed by **one** designated medical practitioner after examination at a psychiatric institution (see definition); may detain the person/patient for a period of **72 hours**.

Form 2   signed by **another** designated medical practitioner after **separate** examination before expiry of 72 hours; shall detain the patient for a period of **one month** for further treatment.

Form 3   signed by **two** designated medical practitioners (**one** of whom shall be a psychiatrist) after **separate** examinations before the expiry of one month; shall detain the patient for further treatment not exceeding **6 months** from the date of the order.

The designated medical practitioners and the psychiatrists who sign such forms should not have **fiduciary** relationship with the patient. A person shall not be detained at a psychiatric institution for treatment unless he is suffering from a **mental disorder**, which then warrants the detention for treatment as it is necessary in the interests of the **health** or **safety** of the person or for the **protection** of other persons that the person should be so detained.

If further detention is required, **Hospital Visitors** shall make an application in accordance with **Form 4** to the **Magistrate**, who may at his discretion sign a detention order in accordance with **Form 5** to extend care and treatment for a period not exceeding **12 months**. During the interim period, the visitors may order by endorsement to detain the patient. Visitors are appointed to inspect the management and condition of the mental hospital and the patients therein at regular intervals of **at least** once every **3 months**.

Sometimes, the police also bring drunkards, vagrants, and illegal immigrants. They should not be admitted if no overt psychotic signs are detected. The more appropriate disposal would be police lock-up, welfare homes, and repatriation respectively.

Normally, the compulsory detention lapses when the "Form" expires on date or when the patient leaves the hospital/institution and is discharged. However, when the patient requires transfer to and treatment in a restructured hospital (RH), arrangements will be made between the Ministry of Law and Ministry of Health to allow the "Form" to be effective and the patient to continue being monitored by IMH routinely. Nurses and doctors must first be informed before receiving RH patients.

C. *Psychiatric Emergencies*

Patients who are **suicidal**, **violent**, or **homicidal** are psychiatric emergencies. The underlying causes may be depression, paranoid disorder, schizophrenic illness, manic psychosis, alcoholism, or drug and personality disorder, just to name some. They should be admitted especially when they have young children or any other vulnerable members in the home. For proper assessment, close kin and friends should be carefully interviewed privately to understand the threat or risk that may be posed by the patients. Past history of similar or recurrent episodes and their management will be very important and useful. Except for those with personality disorders or addictive problems, emergency patients may be referred to the high dependency psychiatric care unit (**HDPCU**) for management. When in doubt, the senior doctor should always be consulted.

On the other hand, we can admit patients for a period of **observation** because of diagnostic difficulty or for inpatient investigation, treatment, and **stabilisation.**

Patients who are **medically ill** and require more extensive investigation and intensive care should be referred to the appropriate general hospitals.

Patients who do not require immediate admission can be observed for up to 23 hours in the special conducive A/E side room under close monitoring. They are provided treatment, counseling, diversion, and psycho-education. An outpatient appointment to see the Department psychiatrist on call is arranged. Admission rate can thus be reduced.

Clerking of Patient

Longitudinal psychiatric assessment spans from "conception to consultation", including maternal health. Clerking should be **systematic** and as **complete** as possible. Any psychopathology would be revealed in due course. Subsequently, significant areas can be focused on, explored, and elaborated. On a busy day, however, the immediate task of the Medical Officer is to determine who should be admitted and to screen patients for any serious medical conditions.

You should develop your own standard procedure. Depending on the circumstances, either the patient or the accompanying person may be interviewed first. It is important to know how long and how well the **informant** has known the patient and whether they have been in contact lately. Do not waste time with informants who are unreliable, subjective, and longwinded.

Interviews are best conducted in the **language** or **dialect** that is **most familiar** to both the doctor and the patient or informant. It is important to always **ascertain** whether what is asked is fully understood and what is answered is equally so. If an interpreter is used, he should be asked to interpret verbatim. When in doubt, do not assume — always **clarify** and **verify**. Questions asked should be purposeful and probing, not haphazard or random. Information recorded should be accurate and factual. The novice should be like a faithful video recorder rather than an impressionistic artist.

An interview may begin with the present complaint or family history depending on the situation and response. If the information is not forthcoming, direct and leading questions may be posed. Patients sometimes prefer to write than to speak.

Technical terms like hallucination, delusion, specific type of thought disorder, and blunted affect are preferably avoided. It is better to write down what is exactly said and observed (e.g., the patient complains of hearing voices talking to or about him and that people want to charm or harm him). If there is no connection, logic, or sense in his talk, give **verbatim** samples rather than concluding that he is irrational, irrelevant, or "thought disordered". Similarly, the mood and manner should also be objectively noted at each point.

Nevertheless, one should know the definition of each technical term clearly, understand what it means, and use it correctly. Different textbooks may have to be referred to.

History Taking

A good history cannot be overemphasised. There is much that can be learned from the past which may shed light on the present. Certain backgrounds tend to shape particular behaviours, and certain personality makeups tend to respond in particular ways. Many mental disorders tend to run a recurrent course. Presence of family history and history of past episodes are of enormous help. **Longitudinal history** in **chronological order** or **developmental sequence** of **events** and **symptoms** is of utmost importance in order to appreciate **primary**, **secondary**, and **chain reactions**. Diagnosis is based on the **primary disturbance** rather than the secondary manifestation or presentation.

Family History

Parents — Age, occupation, health, personality, relationship and marital status (widowed, divorced, remarried, or separated).

If deceased — age and cause of death; any reaction to bereavement; any history of mental illness, alcoholism, suicide, or criminality.

Siblings — Include natural, half, step, adoptive, or fostered.

Birth rank, age, sex, education, occupation, marital status, their relationships, medical history (especially psychiatric).

(Note: **Familial is not synonymous with genetic**)

Household — Nuclear or extended, any in-laws or ill persons; living arrangement, financial state, and atmosphere; any burdens or needed support.

Personal History

Childhood — Birth and milestones, upbringing and caregivers, temperament and behaviour, physical and mental health (e.g., any significant illnesses, operations, hospitalisations, developmental problems, neurotic traits, or conduct disorders); any separation or significant childhood memories and history of abuse.

School — Experience, behaviour, and achievement in primary school (PSLE score), secondary school ("O" levels), junior college ("A" levels, IB etc.), ITE, polytechnic, or tertiary education; extra-curricular activities; any truancy, adverse comments, reports of "beyond parental control", or special commendations.

National Service — Physical employment status, grading, vocation, rank, operationally ready date; any adverse records or coping difficulties; reservist call-up and individual physical proficiency test performance.

Employment — Jobs in chronological order and duration and reason for change; current job and pay; whether coping well and happy with colleagues; if unemployed, for how long and why.

It is important to remember that **work** is an **index of health** and **performance** is related to **wellbeing**. **Inability** to work or deterioration in performance is a sign of **ill health** and its duration can help to date the onset of decompensation or illness.

Psychosexual History

This covers the whole area of psychosexual development, orientation, preference, deviancy (including trans-sexualism, fetishism, and paedophilia), practice, libido, marriage, extramarital relationship, children and family life, serial monogamy, and so on.

Knowledge and experience of sex, masturbatory fantasy, partners, pregnancy and abortion, molest, incest, and rape, when relevant and indicated, ought to be enquired. Note with caution the controversial publicity given to child sexual abuse. First, childhood sexuality differs from adult sexuality. Second, the so-called memory may not be factual. Finally, the link between sexual abuse and psychiatric disorders may be iatrogenic. The question of HIV/AIDS ought to be kept in mind as well as history of exposure and STDs.

Patients who are married should be asked relationship-related questions such as courtship and its duration, age and occupation of spouse, marital relationship, and frequency of intimacy. Information pertaining to sexual intercourse may reveal problems of impotency, frigidity, vaginismus, dyspareunia, obstetric complication, alcoholism, anxiety, delusions of jealousy, hypersexuality from manic state, or loss of libido from depression. It also reflects good or poor marital relationship.

The number, age, and sex of children are also important. They may be a source of stress (e.g., not doing well in school, mixing with wrong company, taking drugs, going out with members of the opposite sex, being addicted to the computer). On the other hand, infertility or not having a male heir can also be a reason for unhappiness.

Financial difficulty and emotional burden, especially in the case of a single parent, should not be overlooked. In extended families, conflict with in-laws is well known.

Problems associated with LGBTQ, sexual gender identity, and dysphoria in our culture is not something people are proud of or will proclaim in public. Therefore, covert homosexuality often presents with disguised or difficult symptoms, which may go on for a long time if the condition is not suspected.

Habits

This would include exercise, drinking, smoking, drug taking, glue sniffing, computer games, internet surfing, and chatting. Note the quantity, frequency, and duration of ingestion or abuse. Identify the substance and the source of supply and determine the cost and effect. Enquire about any associated forensic history or medical complication.

Gambling and debts should be probed. Similar to alcoholism, this is not infrequently the underlying cause of many psychosocial problems. The whole family may be affected and require help.

Premorbid Personality

Information on premorbid personality is most important and yet very difficult to elicit. Premorbid personality refers to before the first onset of illness or during remission between episodes of long-term disorder. The usual answer given by informants is: "He was normal." What we want to know is what sort of a person he was when he was normal or before the change that led him to seek psychiatric help. Without knowing how he was, we will not know how he has changed. The **premorbid baseline** is important for diagnosis, management, and prognosis.

Preferably, the patient is able to tell about himself. He should also be asked what others (e.g., his family members, friends, colleagues, employers) have said of him. He can be asked of his aspirations, values, health, temperament, work, social life, relationships with people, hobbies, religious beliefs, and so on. An account of his **daily routine** may help. He should also be asked whether he has a **nickname** and the reasons for it. It often provides a caricature of his personality. The company he keeps is also a useful clue as "birds of a feather flock together". We need to know the "baseline" when assessing any **abnormal change**. The period of remission in long-term illness may be considered a "baseline".

A "**psychopathological**" approach is often used when information is not forthcoming. Questions may revolve around whether he is an introvert or extrovert, optimist or pessimist, has mood swings, is easily worried or timid, sensitive, suspicious or indifferent, callous, irresponsible, impulsive or meticulous, or indecisive. Is there any history of antisocial behaviour or conduct disorder or past record of offence or conviction? Where available, information from significant others should also be obtained.

Medical History

Past and present medical history should be obtained and their records traced. Hospitalisation, treatment, and medication should be noted. For females, the menstrual history and any associated symptoms should be enquired.

Medical conditions such as head injury, epilepsy, and cardiovascular accidents can have both direct and secondary consequences.

Re-Admissions

For re-admissions, the **social history** of the patient should be **updated**. Changes may provide clues to relapses and affect the management plan. **Changes** include change of home, school, job, leadership, routine, family structure (i.e., due to marriage, birth of a child, divorce or separation, ageing, sickness, death). **Non-compliance** of medication and "**high expressed emotion**" (EE; i.e. **hostility**, **smothering**, **critical** behaviour in the family) are well known factors in relapses. However, "high EE" can also be **induced** by the patient himself/herself.

Interview of Patient

One should endeavour to **know the patient** and **understand his problems** before thinking of making a quick diagnosis.

Routine questions about name, age (DOB), NRIC, address, telephone number, contact person and relatives, day, date, place, reason, and manner brought to hospital help in data collection and building rapport. It also forms part of the mental state examination of orientation, memory, and general intelligence. In addition, organic brain reactions and dementia can more or less be ruled out or established.

Mental State Examination

Mental state examination is actually a **cross-section assessment** of presentation. It should be **descriptive** and **narrative** even as mental state fluctuates and changes. One should keep an **open mind** and not have any preconceived ideas. Remember that the questions asked determine the answers given. Questions should therefore be open-ended.

Objective observations should be **corroborated** by the patient's experience and report before a sign or symptom is firmly established. There is no place for subjective presumption or interpretation, let alone pseudo-authoritative pronouncement. The mnemonics are merely an aid and not to be rigidly adhered to. The signs and symptoms may be congruent, non-congruent, or overlapping.

Appearance

Note the general physical appearance and attire, size, shape, height, weight, complexion, nutritional state, deformity, and posture. Is he old or young for his age? Is he neat and tidy, or disheveled, unkempt, and filthy? Is he overdressed and bizarre, or well-groomed and fashionable? Is he apathetic and self-absorbed, or relaxed and cheerful?

Behaviour

This refers to the overall psychomotor aspect as well as outward expressions of inner experience reflecting one's perception, thinking, and feeling. He may be retarded and withdrawn or excited and agitated. He may stand around and refuse to sit. There may be odd or repeated movements. He may seem distracted and hallucinated or dazed and perplexed. He may be indifferent and mumbling, or talking, smiling, laughing, prying, and gesticulating to himself. He may be resistive, distant, suspicious, and hostile, or co-operative, responsive, and appropriate.

He may be disinhibited, restless, hyperactive, talkative, loud, and over-familiar. He may be anxious, tense, fearful, tearful, and downcast. Some may be timid and shy or childish, silly, and fidgety. Others may appear confused or aggressive.

Conversation

This refers to the manner and content of speech. Talk is a **key to inner thought**, **memory**, **feeling**, and **psychic experience**. Thus, it has been said that: "**So long as the patient talks, we are in business**." When thought is disturbed, speech will be affected. Many forms of thought disorder have been described and there will be various degrees of breakdown in communication. Formal thought disorder refers particularly to that found in schizophrenia, but organic brain lesions, mental retardation, language barriers, and cultural differences must be excluded (see Disorders of Thinking).

To demonstrate thought disorder, verbatim examples of both the questions and the answers should be recorded.

Other aspects to note include speed, flow, direction, linkage, content of speech, and whether the patient thinks his thought is being interfered with. The mind is sometimes crowded with thoughts like a road junction jammed with vehicles because traffic light breakdowns.

Delusion

A delusion is a belief that is **untrue**, **unshakeable**, and **unshared**. The last characteristic may rarely be induced in someone very close to the deluded as in **folie a deux**. Sometimes, what is believed may be a **fact** (e.g., the infidelity of a spouse or partner) and has been described as "**morbid jealousy**" indicating its abnormal or pathological quality. In reality, jealousy may be normal or neurotic in nature or psychotic when it is of clinical and forensic significance. Generally, an acute or abrupt onset due to sudden delusional development is considered a morbid or mono-delusional disorder. Of course, morbid jealousy could also be symptomatic of underlying disorders such as schizophrenia and alcoholism. Difficulty arises when the onset is insidious and the spouse or partner is indeed unfaithful. Nevertheless, with painstaking examination, it is still possible to determine that the factual conclusion has been abnormally derived. The degree or intensity of jealousy does not discriminate between what is normal, neurotic, and psychotic. However, in delusional psychotics, it is the result or nature of disordered thinking.

A delusion may be **primary** or more often **secondary** to hallucinatory experience, mood state, or organic condition. It may be transient or persistent, disorganised or systematised. It is a **psychotic** symptom and depending on the content may be persecutory, grandiose, erotic, or nihilistic. Sometimes, a delusion is very well guarded and hidden and it is a test of interview skill to elicit its presence.

Recovery from delusion may occur in **two stages**. First, the patient stops having active delusions but still maintains that what he had believed earlier on or in the past were true. It is only when he realises that what he had believed in the past were untrue that he has fully recovered. Occasionally, the patient believes that others are abnormal and when he/she improves, he/she would say that others have become better.

Akin to delusional beliefs is the **overvalued idea**. Here, one can understand or sympathise with the overvalued idea held but does not share the complete conviction and commitment in its pursuit. It is a kind of fanaticism.

Emotion

Emotion refers to affect or mood state and relates particularly to **depression** or **elation**. It is not enough to believe or infer that because patients are in low or high spirits, they are suffering from depression or mania. Patients should specifically be asked how they feel and their baseline temperament should be established. In particular, **suicidal thought** and **intent** should be ascertained in the depressed and sad. It is important to determine what is lost and what is the **value** and **meaning** of the "**loss**" to the patient. It is also important to determine who and what there is left to live for. It provides a clue to **suicidal risk**. **Anxiety** and **irritability** are often associated with mood disorders and an attempt ought to be made to distinguish between what is primary and what is secondary.

Fantasy, Factitious, or Fact

It is always important to evaluate and determine what is factual, what is imagination and, what is fabrication. It is also necessary to find out the reasons behind each of these. The **content** and the **motive** are equally informative.

General Knowledge

How well informed is the patient? One should be aware of the going-ons around us (e.g., what is current in the newspapers, TV, radio, internet, and lifestyles of people). The blurring between what is factual and what is fake is rampant nowadays. Educational background and occupational status will more or less indicate one's level of intelligence. If he is mentally retarded/intellectually disabled, he may face difficulties taking care of himself, attending to personal hygiene, telling the date and time, making telephone calls, counting and using money, knowing the bus route and fare, or naming the president.

Hallucination

Hallucinations may be psychotic or non-pathological under certain circumstances. Simply defined, hallucinations are perceptions without real or external stimulus (i.e., not due to voluntary imagination). All sensory modalities can be affected. In pseudo-hallucination, insight is retained. (See Disorders of Perception)

Auditory hallucinations are most frequent. One should ask about their "source", content, effect, and relation to the time of day, sleep, and place. The content of these "voices" is important as the patient may succumb to their instructions and carry out dangerous acts (e.g., homicidal or suicidal behaviour). During recovery, the voices/noises would become softer, further, and less frequent. Patients often complain that voices come from someone or spirits within rather than external to themselves. They may also have difficulty distinguishing what they hear from their own thoughts.

The presence of **olfactory** and **visual** hallucinations may suggest organic conditions whereas **tactile** hallucinations may be due to the passivity phenomenon. In our local population, a positive answer may be more forthcoming if patients are asked about hearing or seeing "dirty" things in their culture (i.e., supernatural or spiritual phenomena which are more acceptable).

Insight

Insight to illness is not easy to ascertain. It is more than the patient's admission or denial of his illness. Awareness and appreciation of loss of wellbeing may be present initially, but the patient may conceal it. Patients with early dementia and schizophrenia may present with depression or anxiety because of initial presence of insight. Compliance with treatment may also indicate insight even if the patient denies illness.

Judgement

Judgement can be very subjective on the part of the observer. Judgement is often retrospective and relative. It involves personal experience, intuition, evaluation, and decision.

Level of Consciousness

It has been said that drowsiness leads to sleep whereas clouding of consciousness leads to coma. Presence and degree of clouding of consciousness as in confusion or delirious states is therefore pathological and indicates central nervous system involvement.

In clouding of consciousness, attention and concentration are affected. The **serial 7** (100 minus 7 consecutively) is generally used to assess attention and concentration. This, however, involves mathematical ability as well. A simpler version of "20 minus 3 consecutively" is also used by some. Alternatively, counting 100 or 20 backward can also be used.

Memory

Complaints of memory loss or poor memory are frequent and associated with fear of brain diseases. The complaint may be objective or subjective. It is necessary to know how memory is formed. (See Disorders of Memory)

Memory function **tests** are objective tests for **organic** lesions of the brain. Broadly, **verbal** memory tests the integrity of the left cerebral hemisphere while **visuo-spatial** memory tests the integrity of the right cerebral hemisphere. A simple clinical test consists of the **ultra short** term (forward and backward digit span), the **short** term (5-minute), and the **long** term (past events). In the short-term memory test, it is important to ensure that the patient has learned what he is to reproduce 5 minutes later by making him repeat it at least once. Numbers, objects, and sentences may be used to remember and reproduce. Another simple test is to ask the patient to draw the face of a clock specifying a time. The patient can also be asked about details of family members or recent events and then go over them again later for reproduction and consistency. In organic conditions, it is the **recent** memory that is first impaired.

Negativism

This may include being unresponsive, resistive, or uncooperative (when instructed to perform activities of daily living) or at times doing exactly the opposite of what is asked. This is in contrast to "automatic obedience" or "command automatism", which is more commonly seen in catatonia and occasionally in dementing conditions.

Orientation

Orientation to person, place, and time should be tested. Orientation to time is usually affected before that of person. During recovery, orientation to person occurs before that of time. Disorientation is a sign of confusion or an organic condition. Some patients may give random answers but are not confused.

Passivity Experience

Passivity experience may be cognitive, affective, volitional, or behavioural. Characteristically, the schizophrenia sufferer complains of being made or compelled to think, feel, or act in specific ways by some external forces. In other words, he is no longer a free agent himself.

Physical Examination

A routine physical examination must always be carried out. Special attention should be paid to evidence of **injuries**, whether external or internal, and must be documented. Protect yourself medico-legally. A quick test of lateralization of neurological signs is useful. Call for more staff to help when the patient is disturbed or violent. Sometimes the patient has to be sedated first and examined later on the ward. An injection of haloperidol 5–10 mg or chlorpromazine 50 mg is also suitable. Others may prefer injection of midazolam or diazepam.

Blood and urine samples should be taken for sugar, alcohol, and drug levels for toxicology when indicated.

Some General Concepts

Problems of Diagnostic Validity

Medical diagnosis ideally should be based on aetiology. However, in mental disorder, aetiology is multifactorial. This is further compounded by the fact that similar conditions or syndromes have been described by different workers in different places and periods of time and given different labels.

Generally speaking, a **diagnostic syndrome** is based on a specific cluster of descriptive symptoms. The **validity** of such a diagnosis is preferably supported by **laboratory investigations**, **family history**, **course and outcome**, **exclusion criteria**, and **therapeutic response** to specific treatments. When all conditions converge or correlate, the validity of the diagnosis is strong.

Common Classes of Mental Disorders (and Related Matters)
Dementias

Dementias are **chronic organic brain syndromes**. When presenting with psychotic symptoms, such as hallucinations, delusional ideation, and abnormal behaviour or superimposed delirious state, they may be regarded as organic psychoses. The **clinical diagnosis** of dementia is based on the **syndrome** of **global deterioration** of **intellect, memory, and personality** (IMP). **Aetiologically**, dementia may be **primary** or **secondary**. Primary dementias consist **chiefly** of Alzheimer's Disease (**AD**) and the more recently highlighted dementias with Lewy bodies (**DLB**) and the frontotemporal lobe. More rare are Pick's, Creutszfeld-Jakob's (which is rapidly dementing), slow virus, or prion diseases in which normal brain protein undergoes conformational change causing the death of brain cells.

Secondary dementias include causes such as multi-infarction of the brain (or vascular dementia, the next most common after AD), head injury, chronic alcoholism, cerebral anoxia, hypothyroidism, neurosyphilis; AIDS, encephalitis, brain tumours, deficiency in vitamins (B12), Huntington's Disease, and Parkinson's Disease. As some causes are reversible, investigation must be thorough and treatment must be vigorous.

Alzheimer's Disease (AD)

As people live longer, the prevalence of dementias, in particular **AD**, will increase rapidly with old age. In **AD**, chromosomes 1, 14, 19, and 21 appear to be implicated with chromosome 19 as responsible for the late onset type. The neurobiological understanding is that there is accumulation (due to overproduction with failure to degrade) of amyloid beta-protein followed by abnormal phosphorylation of tau protein, resulting in massive neuron death in vulnerable brain areas. Senile plaques and neurofibrillary tangles are typically seen in histopathology. Younger age onset is more likely genetic.

The clinical course of progressive or degenerative **primary dementias** such as **AD** may be divided into three phases:

1. **Psychological** — the disease may initially present with anxiety and depression, forgetfulness, (disorientation), accentuation of personal traits or erratic behaviours that are out of character, and symptoms of delusion and hallucination. The onset may be insidious.
2. **Neurological** — motor restlessness, dysarthria or aphasia, dysphagia, apraxia, slow mentation, abnormal reflexes, poor coordination, ataxia and seizures, etc.
3. **Vegetative** — loss of memory, speech, social interaction, and personal identity. The patient eventually becomes bed ridden, incontinent, and totally dependent.

Biomarkers of AD

Compared with other dementing disorders, tau protein in **cerebrospinal fluid** (CSF) is significantly increased in AD. The tau level is not correlated with duration of the disease or score on the mini mental state examination (MMSE). On the other hand, beta-amyloid-42 protein is significantly decreased because in advanced AD, the insoluble beta-amyloid attracts the soluble beta-amyloid and locks it up. In mild cognitive impairment (**MCI**) or very early stage dementia, tau is increased but beta-amyloid is normal. Perhaps it can be predicted that during the transition of MCI to AD, beta-amyloid in CSF would decrease. Thus, a combined measure of tau protein and beta-amyloid protein is a better marker for AD, demonstrating more than 85% of sensitivity and specificity. It is highly sensitive in differentiating early and incipient AD from normal ageing, depression, alcohol dementia, and Parkinson's disease, but has lower specificity against other dementias (i.e., frontotemporal and Lewy body dementia). This is important for the evaluation of MCI and earlier detection of the clinical stage of dementia and AD.

Approximately 10% to 30% of individuals who are clinically diagnosed with AD do not display neuropathologic changes associated with AD at autopsy or have normal findings in amyloid positron-emission tomography (PET) or CSF $A\beta_{42}$ studies (indicating the possibility of wrong diagnosis).

Conversely, neuropathologic changes associated with AD can be present without signs or symptoms. Thirty percent to 40% of cognitively unimpaired individuals are found to have neuropathologic changes at autopsy or abnormal amyloid biomarkers (indicating the possibility of missed diagnosis).

Biological Treatment and Psychosocial Intervention

Therapeutic approaches depend on different pathophysiological hypotheses or beta amyloidogenic pathways requiring different mechanistic markers.

There is active research that is both biological and psychosocial on pathogenesis, prevention, and treatment of AD. These include:

1. Gamma-secretase inhibition
2. Metal-protein attenuating compounds (MPACs)
3. Immunisation with beta-amyloid
4. Cholesterol metabolism
   Lowering cerebral cholesterol may decrease beta-amyloid production possibly through the beta-secretase pathway. Prospective studies with statins are being actively investigated.
5. Beta-amyloid binding proteins (in vivo) e.g. glycosaminoglycan may inhibit fibrillization.
6. Other investigated agents in trials include NMDA antagonists, ampakines, anti-amyloid strategies, anti-inflammatory agents, chelators, gingko, and hormones.
7. **Insulin** is a neurotrophic factor with a major role in inhibiting apoptosis or cell death. It may be critical to normal brain circuitry. Yet, about 10–20% of AD are estimated to be the result of diabetes. Both diabetes and obesity increase the risk of MCI and likewise depression. Amyloid has pro-inflammatory and insulin-resistant effects. [Roger Mcintyre]

   Lithium is being investigated for its protection of nerve cells by preventing the phosphorylation of tau protein that is essential to normal brain function but harmful when in excess, resulting in cell death and dementia.
8. There is also increasing data on the efficacy of antidepressants and anti-psychotics for treating specific behaviours in dementia. They can stimulate the brain-derived neurotrophic factor (BDNF).
9. Psychosocial intervention includes a generally healthy lifestyle of good dietary habits, exercise, satisfactory interpersonal relationships, music, reading, and so on.

Cholinesterase inhibitors represent the first approved strategy for treating AD. The rationale is that there is a deficit of acetylcholine neurotransmitters from damage to an ascending forebrain projection. There are also trials on combinations of the cholinesterase inhibitor with a variety of agents (glutamate antagonists, sertraline, risperidone, vitamins, and statins).

Although Lewy bodies are also found in other dementias, **DLB** characteristically presents with auditory and visual hallucinations, Parkinsonism, and fluctuating cognitive impairment besides symptoms of dementia. There is neuroleptic sensitivity (i.e., worsened by drugs with anticholinergic side effects). In Parkinson's Disease, at least 25–30% or more cumulatively will become demented. However, dementing symptoms are said to develop more than 12 months after initial motor symptoms and should therefore be diagnosed as Parkinson's Disease Dementia (PDD). Management of dementias depends on the stage of the illness diagnosed and the symptoms complained of. Of course, psychosocial factors and behavioural approaches cannot be ignored. (See section on Psychogeriatrics)

Psychosis

Concept of Psychosis

A) **Phenomenology** — Phenomenologically, the traditional definition of psychosis is a mental condition in which the signs and symptoms are:

> **Non-understandable** (in ordinary sense of thought, speech, and behaviour)
>
> **Out of touch with reality** (alien to cultural context of mores and norms)
>
> **No insight** (that is contextual and relative)

B) **Social/Lay Madness** — due to **breakdown** in **cultural…:**

Conformity — "communal context" (but spirit possession and trance state accepted)

Communication — "interpersonal context" (not due to IQ, language barrier, culture)

Control — "individual context" (in response to abnormal psychic experience)

Thus, the appearance and behaviour may be bizarre, intolerable, and unacceptable, the speech may be incoherent, irrational, and irrelevant, and as a result of abnormal experience and belief, the psychotic may act out beyond self-control.

Reports or history of having consulted temple **mediums** or **deities** or **bomohs** suggest psychotic disturbance. It is worthwhile to enquire what has transpired and what the healer actually says. Cultural beliefs are powerful and can undermine or facilitate medical treatment.

C) **Clinical Psychoses** — based on presence of one or more psychopathologies or symptoms of:

Hallucination, Delusion, Thought Disorder, Abnormal Mood, Anomalous Behaviour or **Movement, Loss of Volition/Drive, Passivity Experience** (loss of autonomy and control; i.e., made to think, feel, and do)

(to be differentiated from thought disorder, mood disorder, and compulsive behaviour)

Symptoms may be primary or secondary e.g. primary hallucination and secondary delusion

Contents may or may not be offensive or dangerous or acted upon.

Traditionally, **Schizophrenia** and **Manic-Depressive Psychosis** (now **Bipolar Disorders**) have been considered as **typical psychoses** and other primary psychotic disorders (e.g., schizoaffective psychosis) are considered **atypical psychoses.**

D) Medico-legal Insanity (or Unsoundness of Mind)

"Unsoundness of mind" or **legal insanity** is not the same as **medical psychosis**. In other words, clinical psychosis need not be legally insane or of unsound mind whereas mental retardation or intellectual disability without psychosis may qualify (see below).

There are different **connotations** in different **contexts** of the **Penal Code, Criminal Procedure Code**, and the **Mental Health (Care and Treatment) Act (MHCTA-2008)** as well as in **Civil Laws**. A person may be unsound in one context and yet not unsound in another. In general, it involves assessment of issues regarding **credibility, culpability, competency, compensation**, and **custody (Slovenko).** Although the term "**unsound mind**" is not defined, in normal understanding, it consists of **two components** — presence of a **mental disorder** (psychosis or mental retardation/intellectual disability as in our practice) that is **essential** and **consequential** to satisfying the **set of criteria or tests** pertaining to the legal issue in question (e.g., fitness to plead, criminal responsibility, testamentary capacity, property transaction, marriage contract, custody of child, detention for treatment, and appointment of committee(s) of the person and/or his estate, etc). However, in reality, the legal set of criteria or tests appears to **dominate the determination of** soundness or unsoundness of mind. As such, the **causative factor** of "defect of reason from disease of the mind" is not confined to that of a mental disorder but logically includes **disease of the brain**. The final decision lies with the court.

The Mental Health (Care and Treatment) Act [MHCTA] 2008 and the Mental Capacity Act [MCA] 2008, which repeal MDTA (1985), do not use "unsoundness of mind". Instead, mental disorder or the mentally disordered are mentioned and made more explicit to include psychiatric illness, learning disability, dementia, or brain damage that impair or disturb the functioning of the mind or brain. MHCTA provides for the detention, care, and treatment of mentally disordered persons in designated psychiatric institutions. MCA deals with the assessment of persons who lack the capacity to make decisions and take action, among other matters.

(See Chapter 7 on Law and Psychiatry)   14 May 2019

Neuroses

It is often taught that neuroses differ from psychoses in that the symptoms (e.g., fear, sadness, fastidiousness) are understandable, the individual is in contact with reality, and there is presence of insight. Although these criteria are not absolute clinically, they indicate that the feelings and reactions of neurotic states are **common** and **shared** by normal people as well. What separates neurotic complaints from the ordinary are the **intensity**, **duration**, and **frequency** of the symptoms. This of course does not preclude the psychopathological basis of neurotic disorders (see Neurotic and Stress-Related Disorders, and Treatment of Neuroses).

Somatic Symptom and Related Disorders — DSM-5

Disorders of bodily distress or bodily experience — ICD-11

Somatic symptom and related disorders have replaced the somatoform disorder diagnoses of DSM-IV. In this group of disorders, the common feature is the prominence of somatic symptoms associated with significant **distress** and **impairment**. They may occur in mental or medical settings and overcome the old "psychosomatic" concept indicating apparent absence of medical explanations for physical symptoms and their secondary effects.

The classical "psycho-physiological" or "psychosomatic" disorders (e.g., asthma, peptic ulcers, headache) emphasise psychogenic aetiology, which has been found to be unsatisfactory. The objection is that this view encourages the splitting of mind and body. Thus, the **World Health Organization (1964)** stresses a **holistic** approach to medicine and to all diseases in its statement: "When we speak of psychological processes and physiological processes we are speaking of different ways of approaching one phenomenon. The phenomenon is not so divided." Psychosomatic medicine should therefore denote holistic medicine.

In fact, long ago, **Plato** had said: "This is the great error of our day in the treatment of the human body that physicians separate the soul from the body. The cure of a part should not be attempted without treatment of the whole. No attempt should be made to cure the body without the soul and if the head and body are to be healthy you must begin by curing the mind."

To avoid the dichotomy of body and mind, purely descriptive terms are coined for these various, multiple, recurrent, and/ or changing physical symptoms which have no discovered organic basis. Although no aetiology is offered, it does not mean **emotional conflict** and **psychological stress** are to be ignored.

In **DSM-5**, somatic symptom and related disorders include somatic symptom disorder, illness anxiety disorder, conversion disorder, psychological factors affecting other medical conditions, factitious disorder, and other specified or unspecified somatic symptom and related disorders. **Dissociative** (conversion) disorders are new terms for old **hysteria.**

In **ICD-11, dissociative disorders** exist separately from **disorders of bodily distress or bodily experience** and include both conversion (somatic) symptoms and dissociative phenomena, such as amnesia, fugue, or trance state and so-called multiple personality disorder. Here again, **bodily distress disorder** excludes Tourette's syndrome and tics, hair pulling and plucking, hypochondriasis, body dysmorphic disorder, and excoriation disorder.

In **hysteria** (conversion and dissociation), the symptoms are unconsciously produced with unconscious purpose. In **factitious disorder**, the symptoms are consciously produced but with unconscious motives. In **malingering**, the symptoms are consciously produced with conscious motives.

Body dysmorphic disorder (BDD) appears to straddle across hypochondriacal or somatic symptom disorder and delusional or psychotic disorder. However, in DSM-5, it is grouped under obsessive-compulsive disorder together with hoarding disorder, trichotillomania, and excoriation disorder.

Generally speaking, respiration, circulation, digestion, nerve conduction, muscle contraction, and even the sensorium **function continuously** in **self-monitoring without our awareness**. However, we become conscious of morbidity only when **malfunctioning** occurs. It is also possible that we become **sensitised** to what is going on in certain parts of our body by **heightened attention** or **lowered threshold** of sensation. It is like the naked eye that sees nothing on a slide, but when a portion is focused under the microscope, details are magnified and seen clearly. Similarly, there are all sorts of radio and television waves around us which "come alive" in sound and picture only when tuned in.

Personality Disorder(s)

Personality may be regarded as the sum total of an individual's physical endowment, mental capacity, emotional experience, and pattern of behavioural response. Together, they manifest certain **traits** and **tendencies** that are enduring, predictable, and evident from young. Self-identity and esteem, interpersonal relationships, family and social roles, education, occupation, and other functional roles are all involved. These traits and tendencies may be an advantage or disadvantage depending on the circumstances. However, some traits and tendencies, when excessive and non-adaptive, become a liability and cause distress, difficulty, and disturbance in self-image, relationships, work, and social conduct. Not only does the individual himself or herself suffer, but others and society at large may also be affected. When this is persistent, a personality disturbance or disorder is said to exist.

The classification of personality disorders has been **controversial** and **in a state of flux**. In **ICD-11**, existing categories of personality disorder from ICD-10 reflecting specific traits or patterns of behaviour are removed and replaced by a main and "generic" personality disorder classified as mild, moderate, or severe. Prominent personality traits or patterns of domain qualifiers may be in a continuum from normal to dominant/disturbed and subsumed under personality disorder. "**Mild**" indicates disturbance in some areas of functioning and typically does not cause harm to self or others. "**Moderate**" affects multiple areas of functioning and may be associated with harm to self and others. In "**severe**", most if not all areas of personality functioning are affected with interpersonal disturbance and are associated with harm to self and others. Other categories of personality disorder or personality difficulty include negative affectivity, detachment, dissociality (or antisociality), disinhibition, anankastic personality (rigid perfectionism), and borderline behaviour patterns (of instability, impulsivity, emptiness, and self-harm). In sum, **personality dysfunction** is best represented on a **continuum** or **dimension** with **different levels of severity** of personality functioning at the time of assessment, including the relatively recent past. The severity of personality disturbance ranges from no personality **dysfunction** to personality **difficulty** (not a disorder) to mild, moderate, and severe personality **disorder**. [Peter Tyrer]

However, in current clinical and forensic settings, diagnosis of a personality problem/difficulty/disorder is often based on "**trait symptoms**" and "**behavioural patterns**" over a prolonged period of time. The significance of these personality problems, difficulties, or disorders is that they are of clinical and forensic interest with regard to **capability**, **suffering**, and **criminal responsibility**, respectively. The implication is that such conditions are "medical" in nature and therefore amenable to treatment. This is in contrast to the concept of stable personality traits in psychology. However, people do seem to change (at least behaviourally) as a result of diseases (e.g., brain-damage and encephalitis or life experiences and psychotherapy), which can set off a series of chain reactions. It is important to remember and recognise personality factors in any management. Nonetheless, the term "**borderline personality**" is often overused and diagnosed without clear understanding of its historical development and domains involved.

Life Events

Life events are **significant** experiences that occur during an individual's lifetime. They may vary from society to society and from one period of time to another. Some common life events include birth, coming of age, school enrolment, examinations, starting a new job, promotion, unemployment, marriage, divorce, moving house, illness, retirement, death, birthdays, anniversaries, and festive celebrations. The **quantum** of significance of each life event **varies** with each individual and at different stages of life.

Life events bring about **changes** or **threats** that require the individual to exert **effort to adjust** or **cope**. They are like stressors that can cause distress and precipitate or exacerbate illnesses. The same life event may cause different symptoms in different persons with variable consequences. It is not unlike the same bacteria that can cause different diseases in different organs in the body.

Epilepsy

Epileptic phenomena are truly neuropsychiatric problems. Epileptic seizures are recurrent paroxysmal electrical discharges from focal lesions in the brain. **Focal** (or localised or partial) seizures may arise from a part of the brain (i.e., the frontal, temporal, parietal, or occipital lobe). It is called a **simple partial seizure** when restricted with **no loss of consciousness**. When the discharge spreads to other parts of the brain or the whole cerebral hemisphere with possible loss of consciousness, it is called a **complex partial seizure** (as in **temporal lobe epilepsy** or psychomotor seizures). The **prodromal** simple partial seizure is then known as an **aura**. In **generalised seizures**, both the cerebral hemispheres are involved as in generalised motor seizures (grand mal fits) and **absence** seizures (petit mal fits) with **loss of consciousness**. In the 18th Edition of Harrison's Internal Medicine (2011), partial seizures are divided into "**partial seizures with dyscognitive features**" and "**partial seizures without dyscognitive features**".

The type of seizure observed or reported depends on the direction, extent, and speed of discharge from the focal lesion. Thus, epileptic seizures may be motor (e.g., convulsions or involuntary movements), sensory (e.g., sensations and hallucinations), autonomic (e.g., nausea, palpitation, sweating, flushing), affective (e.g., fear, anger, depression), psychic (e.g., déjà vu, flashing images), and behavioural (e.g., automatism without awareness) either alone or in combination. In partial seizures, the symptoms vary according to the site of discharge and the subjective content. **They may mimic psychiatric disorders**.

The typical history is that there may be birth injuries and/ or childhood (febrile) seizures that go into remission. After a prolonged latent period, seizures appear in adolescence and can present with grand mal, petit mal, and psychomotor attacks on different occasions or in combination.

Recurrence of paroxysmal and stereotyped sequential progress of symptoms must be established. Amnesia follows when there is unawareness or loss of consciousness. It must be emphasised that diagnosis of epilepsy is based on clinical history.

"**Epileptic psychosis**" refers to psychotic manifestations associated with epileptic seizures. **Temporally**, it may be **prodromal**, **ictal**, **post-ictal**, or **inter-ictal**. **Clinically**, it may be **organic** (ictal/post-ictal confusion) or **functional** (inter-ictal schizophrenia-like symptoms) in nature. Personality change may be involved as a result of brain dysfunction, prolonged medication, and chain reaction in psychosocial development.

Drug-Induced Psychosis

With more and more drugs of abuse available, it has become important to recognise their effects on the mind and behaviour. Some mental symptoms occur during states of intoxication and some during the stages of withdrawal. Depending on the property of the drug, the mental makeup

of the user, and the immediate surrounding environment, consciousness, perception, and mood state are variably altered with matching behaviour. The experience may be pleasant or unpleasant and paradoxical reactions are not uncommon (e.g., in benzodiazepines).

Acute intoxication may result in acute brain syndrome while chronic use may result in chronic brain syndrome. The prolonged use of a drug may lead to **tolerance** and **dependency**. In tolerance, the user needs to take more and more of the drug to achieve or attain the same desired effects. Dependency may be physical due to withdrawal symptoms or psychological when there is emotional and mental preoccupation with the drug's effects and a persistent craving for the drug.

When psychotic symptoms occur as a result of drug taking, then a diagnosis of **"drug-induced psychosis"** is made. There has been much debate on the concept of "drug-induced psychosis". The difficulty seems to be that the term "induced" is used in both the **aetiological** and **precipitating** sense. If the psychotic symptoms are limited **temporally** according to the **presence** and **action** of the substance used (e.g., in bupropion), then "induced" may have the aetiological meaning. On the other hand, if the psychotic symptoms persist beyond the temporal presence and action of the substance used, then "induced" would mean precipitating. However, it is difficult to demonstrate the nature of either condition as brain damage with lasting symptoms can be caused by drugs such as **methamphetamine** (MAMP) and some inhalants. Early and prolonged use of methamphetamine has been associated with increased risk of psychosis similar to the positive symptoms of schizophrenia in vulnerable personality (schizoid/schizotypal?). Amphetamine use may cause short term (during intoxication and withdrawal schizophrenic symptoms). Heavy early use of **cannabis** probably exerts its effect via the dopamine system, which is moderated by a genetic polymorphism in catechol-O-methyltransferase (COMT) that reduces frontal cortex dopamine transmission of the susceptible to induce schizophreniform psychosis. As such, it has a **predisposing** sense in inducing psychosis.

Assessment of "Dangerousness" or Risk and Suicide

Dangerousness

Not infrequently, one is asked to predict the "**dangerousness**" of a person. More specifically, the request should be to assess the "**risk**" of dangerous behaviour or response by a particular individual in a particular situation at a particular time. In other words, the so-called dangerousness of a person should be **context specific**. Thus, to be meaningful, both the patient's mental state or condition and prevailing environmental circumstances must be assessed together in context. A past history of dangerous behaviour would be a good predictor.

The following factors should be considered when making an assessment:

Inherent aggression or impulsivity directed at self or others due to personality traits or cultural upbringing, conduct/personality disorder, or genetic makeup

Symptomatic behaviour of underlying brain disease or mental disorder (e.g., epilepsy, alcohol use, drug use, affective and schizophrenic disorders)

Interactive with or in response to environmental factors (e.g., provocation, threat, stress)

Suicide

There are many explanations or reasons why people commit suicide. Many are mentally and physically ill or socially distressed while some are not. A few may give no indication whatsoever of their suicidal intent until it happens.

People may kill themselves because they are depressed and distressed; in response to command hallucinations, passivity experience, or persecutory delusions; because of insight of prognosis; under the influence of drug and alcohol; or because of personality problems.

There are many schedules for assessment of suicidal risk. A most important risk is when there is nothing — not even immediate loved ones — to live for and there is no religious or spiritual belief or anchor. Although attempted suicide has been regarded as an offence, it is being decriminalised.

Approach to Diagnosis

It is important to realise that for every piece of behaviour (e.g., violence), there can be a number of reasons or explanations, and for every complaint or symptom (e.g., insomnia), there can be a variety of diagnoses. In diagnosis, one should not adopt a checklist approach to "what" the symptoms are but rather consider the whole clinical picture of "why" and "when" in development. The question of "what are the facts of the case?", especially in forensic practice, must always be asked and determined. The following steps may be helpful:

1. The first question to ask is whether there is a normal (or abnormal) and understandable (or non-understandable) change.

When there is an abnormal change (i.e., departure from the norm or premorbid baseline of behavioural pattern and daily routines), there will be impaired well-being, psychosocial function, work performance, or unemployment indicating onset of illness.

2. Abnormal and non-understandable change is likely to be due to psychosis.

3. If psychotic, is it organic, schizophrenic, affective, or delusional?

4. Is the change acute or chronic (e.g., delirium or dementia)? Substance abuse disorders presenting with a state of confusion may be due to intoxication or withdrawal.

   (Many delusional symptoms may have underlying organic conditions.)

5. When the change is understandable, due to an exogenous reaction (i.e., due to stress), the complaints (e.g., worry, fear, sadness) are out of proportion in intensity, duration, and frequency, and psychosocial functioning is affected, *"neurotic"* conditions are likely.

   (However, when patients present with "inexplicable" withdrawal or fearfulness, early schizophrenia/psychosis ought to be excluded.)

6. Remember to think of the underlying personality and to always exclude temporal lobe epilepsy, history of encephalitis, frontal lobe syndrome (e.g., appearing clinically depressed and retarded or antisocial and disinhibited), hypo/hyperthyroidism, effects of alcohol and drugs, HIV/AIDS, and autoimmune/inflammatory disease.

7. Is there a past similar episode and treatment and family history?

Different persons at distinct stages of life react to the same illness differently. The interaction between personality traits and symptoms or the superimposition of one disorder on another can make diagnosis difficult. Bipolar and schizoaffective disorders are often retrospective from reviewing patients' past longitudinal history of episodes and presentations. Different diagnoses may be arrived at by different clinicians who examine the patient at different time points during the illness. It is important to keep in mind that the patient should not be made to fit a diagnosis (from a checklist of symptoms or out of convenience), but rather the most appropriate diagnosis is selected to fit the patient. Management is then tailored according to the total needs of the individual patient and not treatment of his diagnosis per se.

There have been expanding categories and classifications of mental disorders and changes in concepts, definitions, criteria, and nomenclature in each updated edition or revision of the ICD and DSM. As such, the matter is still in flux and not static. Not all mental conditions are diagnosable by the ICD/DSM and may be termed "unspecified" or classified elsewhere.

Chapter 4
Common Mental Disorders

The diagnosis of a mental disorder, in the absence of known aetiology or mechanism, depends on **symptom cluster** and (arbitrary) **duration** criteria. This is usually decided by consensus of opinion rather than by nosological concept. There is also the question of whether one takes a longitudinal (historical course) or cross-sectional (episodic) view. Some disorders such as "**schizotypal**", "**dysthymic**", and "**cyclothymic**" may be considered "sub-threshold" or "attenuated" forms of major schizophrenic and affective disorders over long periods.

Due to developmental and conceptual changes, some mental disorders are considered categorical entities while others are seen as dimensional; that is, in a continuum or spectrum. Thus, schizophrenia and manic-depressive psychosis (bipolar disorder) had initially been categorical entities but were later argued to be dimensional and occupying opposite ends of a continuum/spectrum with schizoaffective disorder in between. The evidence seems to indicate that there is some overlapping of shared genes. In similar fashion, Asperger's disease has become part of the autism spectrum disorders. Likewise, depression, anxiety, phobias, and OCD (though separate now) may be similarly linked. However, schizophrenia (and primary psychotic disorders), bipolar and related disorders, and mood disorders stand separately, though they are connected.

[See ICD-11 on Mental, behavioural or neurodevelopmental diorders.]

Schizophrenia

Schizophrenia is a generic term for a **heterogeneous** syndrome or other primary psychotic disorders. The pathogenesis and epigenesis as well as pathophysiology and psychopathology are complex and neurodevelopmental in concept and involve psychosocial factors as well. The classifications are not final because of myriad variations. In **ICD-11**, the types of **schizophrenia** are classified or coded according to episode, recovery/remission, and course.

First Episode — currently symptomatic, in partial remission, in full remission

Multiple Episodes — currently symptomatic, in partial remission, in full remission

Continuous — currently symptomatic, in partial remission, in full remission

Meanwhile, according to the **ICD-10 (1992)**, schizophrenic disorders exhibit some of the following symptoms for a period of **one month**:

1. **Thought** — Echo (hearing one's own thoughts as voices), Insertion, Withdrawal, Broadcasting (which is particularly distressing because of the loss of control and privacy over one's own thoughts), and Thought Block when thought comes to a halt (i.e., Schneider's First Rank).
2. Delusions of control, influence, or **Passivity** — affecting action, sensation, or thought. Here, the patient complains of being made to think, feel, do, or behave in certain ways.

3. **Hallucinatory voices** — Running Commentary (commenting on the patient's every action and movement), Discussing the patient in the third person (i.e., Schneider's First Rank)

   Command hallucinations — telling the patient what to do which can be dangerous and disastrous (e.g., "voices" from parts of the body)
4. **Persistent Delusions** — Untrue, Unshared, and Unshakeable beliefs (e.g., aliens and the supernatural) that develop suddenly or gradually.
5. **Persistent Hallucinations** — Any modality, but especially auditory.
6. **Thought Disorder** — Breakdown in communication not due to organic lesions, mental retardation, language barriers, or cultural differences (see Disorders in Thinking). May be random, disinhibited, direct, intrusive, personal, and uncensored.
7. **Catatonic Behaviour** — Stupor or Excitement, Waxy Flexibility, Posturing, Negativism, Mutism (**Catatonia** also exists as a separate disorder category).
8. **"Negative" symptoms** — Social Withdrawal, Poverty of Speech, Loss of Volition, Blunting of Affect, Psychomotor Retardation.
9. **Overall deterioration** and change in quality of life and behaviour (e.g., apathy, indolence, self-neglect, social drifting, or withdrawal).

Schizophrenic disorders have been classified according to the most prominent symptoms or combinations of symptoms/features exhibited (i.e., **paranoid, catatonic, hebephrenic, undifferentiated, residual or simple**). In **Delusional Disorders**, the symptoms are chiefly delusional. The core deficit of schizophrenia appears to be **cognitive impairment** affecting executive functions. These are similar to Emil Kraepelin's (1899) chronic, deteriorating "dementia precox" and what **E. Bleuler** (1911) describes as the central psychopathology of schizophrenia (i.e., loosening of **association** in thinking, blunting of **affect, autism** or withdrawal behaviour, and **ambivalence** or weakening of volition/ will). Bleuler considers **hallucination** and **delusion** as **accessory** symptoms. It is noteworthy that in clinical practice, we rely heavily on the presence of auditory hallucinations and delusional ideas as described by Kurt Schneider's '**First-Rank Symptoms**' (1938) to form a diagnosis of schizophrenia. These symptoms are, however, not pathognomonic and their diagnostic significance is under review (e.g., normal persons without psychosis may exhibit thought disorder). They have also been described in the symptomatology of bipolar disorders.

Crow and Andreasen (1980s) — describe two syndromes of schizophrenia:

Positive symptoms: Hallucinations, delusions, thought disorder +/– inappropriate affect, abnormal behaviour

Negative symptoms (not absence of symptoms): Poverty of speech, loss of volition, psychomotor retardation, social withdrawal, blunting of affect. (They may be of primary insidious onset or due to burnt out end stage, or secondary to medication.)

During the early stages, positive symptoms may be prominent and dominate. As the illness progresses, negative symptoms may become more apparent and dominant eventually.

Pathogenesis

From **family, adoption**, and **twin studies, biological factors** are well established. Thus, the closer the blood relations and the greater the number of family members afflicted, the higher the probability of offspring developing the illness. However, the fact that **monozygotic** twins (i.e., siblings with the same genetic makeup) do **not** show a 100% concordance rate indicates that other factors are also involved. In fact, one twin could suffer from schizophrenia and the other a bipolar disorder. It has been suggested that the earlier the onset, the more likely it is due to genetic and developmental factors. However, it would also be correct to say that both genetic and environmental factors contribute to the development of schizophrenia.

Genetically, the presence of susceptible genes, including neuregulin 1 (in chromosome 8p), dysbindin (chromosome 6p), and catechol-O-methyltransferase (chromosome 22q) in normal variation, may predispose individuals with childhood abnormalities such as delayed motor development (particularly walking), speech problems, lower IQ, and social anxiety to develop schizophrenia. Other hypothesised factors include **birth injuries** and viral **infections** that manifest their effects during critical neurodevelopmental stages. However, research in recent years shows that patients with schizophrenia have severe impaired neuroplasticity or "synaptopathy" (i.e., downregulation of synaptic proteins/disturbance of micro-connectivity) and brain volume decrement from white matter rather than grey matter. This neurodegeneration is associated with decline in growth factors. A combined neurodevelopmental and neurodegenerative model is therefore possible.

Social theories on patterns of parenting, migration, poverty, and stress are also advocated.

Taking the average of various studies, the prevalence of schizophrenia in a population is about 0.5–1%; the risk in first-degree relatives is 10% or more and in identical twins 40% or more. In general, it can be said that genetics contribute 70% while environmental factors account for 30% to the cause of the disease.

Pathophysiology

The current dominant **Dopamine Hypothesis** postulates that the "positive" psychotic symptoms in schizophrenia are due to hyper-dopaminergic activity in the brain (i.e., the mesolimbic pathway or system) while the "negative" symptoms are due to hypo-dopaminergic activity in the mesocortical pathway or system. The support for this hypothesis comes from the efficacy of antipsychotic drugs that are mainly dopamine antagonists or relative agonists to the receptors. Other psychotogenic pathways may be due to glutamate excitotoxicity, such as stimulation of NMDA (N-methyl-D-aspartate) receptors, GABA dysfunction linked to 5HT receptors, and oxidative stress, which lead to reduction in neurogenesis (see Chapter 5).

Schizophrenia, meaning **splitting** of the mind, was coined by **E. Bleuler** (1911) to describe the breaking up of the mental functions. As mentioned before, different aspects of mental functions are interrelated, interactive, and integrated. In diseased conditions of the mind or brain, these functions undergo **variable** and **differential dissociation, disorganization, disintegration,** and **regression,** thereby affecting part or all of the individual's psychic experience, behavioural responses, and social functioning. The effects may vary from mild and subtle cognitive deficits to complete fragmentation and incongruity of mental functions. The clinical spectrum may range from oddities of speech and habit, lack of productivity, and deterioration of performance to obvious psychotic breakdown with recognised core features. In recent years, **Japanese** psychiatrists have used the term "**Integration Disorder**" in place of schizophrenia, which has become stigmatising. Results show that patients and families are more willing to come for early consultation and are more compliant in treatment.

The patient may exert control and conceal his hallucinations and delusions or, if not, talk back to "voices" and attack his "persecutor"; he may hide in fear from imagined harm, avoid "poisonous" food, and withdraw from others. He may laugh and cry without apparent reason, behave oddly without being self-conscious, or become childish and incoherent. In a chronic state, he may appear lazy, unkempt, and shabby. Often, he withdraws from others or avoids crowds to protect himself from over-arousal or stimulation which overwhelms him. When overexposed, his mind gets "jammed up" and he experiences great intrapsychic anxiety with tachycardia. It is like clicking the mouse repeatedly and rapidly, causing the CPU to be unable to respond accordingly and the process is delayed or hangs. A break, rest, or even rebooting is necessary for functions to be restored. It helps for schizophrenic patients to have inter-mittent respite when they feel that their mind is "overcrowded" or stressed.

Schizoaffective Disorders

The concepts and definitions of schizoaffective disorders have been confusing and controversial. Nevertheless, according to ICD-10 as well as ICD-11: "These are episodic disorders in which both affective and schizophrenic symptoms are prominent within the same episode of illness, preferably simultaneously, but at least within a few days of each other." Patients who have been diag-nosed to suffer from schizoaffective disorders often have an initial florid and undifferentiated psychotic episode during adolescence. The clinical picture is one of mixed organic, schizophrenic, and affective features. However, with time, the psychosis may become more differentiated and the patient may subsequently show only schizophrenic, affective, or mixed symptoms in other episodes. Precipitating stressors are commonly present. It is not unlike tem-poral lobe epilepsy, frequently with a past history of childhood febrile fit, which later may present with variable seizures such as psychomotor, grand mal, and petit mal attacks depending on the direction, speed, and extent of discharge from the focal lesion. In DSM-5, schizoaffective disorder can be diagnosed when there are mixed affective and schizophrenic episodes occurring in the longitudinal history.

Schizoaffective disorder is similarly classified as first episode, multiple episodes, or continuous — currently symptomatic, in partial remission, or in full remission.

It is noteworthy that there is some similarity between manic hyperactivity or stupor and catatonic excitement or stupor, which may be due to hyper-dopaminergic activity. There is also some similarity between depression with psychomotor retardation and schizophrenia with negative symptoms, which may also be due to hypo-dopaminergic activity. Differential gradient of dopaminergic activity and interaction between the different pathways may result in production of different symptoms or syndromes.

Robin Murray (Institute of Psychiatry — London)

Robin Murray is of the opinion that the Kraepelinian dichotomy of distinct schizophrenia and bipolar disorders are actually part of the **same continuum** in which bipolar patients experience psychosis and schizophrenic patients experience depression or manic episodes. They not only **overlap in symptoms** but also have onset in early adulthood and respond to dopamine blockade. Thus, in monozygotic twins, they are more likely to develop the same illness and are also more at risk of exhibiting symptoms of the other illness because they **share certain susceptible genes** for psychosis, such as neuregulin 1, dysbidin, and COMT. However, those who suffer from bipolar disorders tend to be spared impediment in intellectual development and education and have better outcomes while being sensitive to major life events. Schizophrenia tends to result in more severe cognitive impairment and poorer outcomes. Therefore, schizophrenia comprises **five syndromes: positive** symptoms, **negative** symptoms, **manic** episodes, **depression**, and **disorganization**. Besides psychotic symptoms, associated affective and anxiety symptoms also need to be treated as they may help to prevent onset of psychosis. There is also an important role for cognitive behavioural therapy (i.e., in areas of cognitive deficits; see Anxiety is the "Mother of Psychopathology").

Affective (Mood) Disorders

Affect, mood, emotion, and feeling have been defined and used differently in different textbooks. However, in clinical practice, "affect" and "mood" are interchangeable terms. Mood disorders in ICD-11 include depressive episodes, manic episodes, mixed episodes, and hypomanic episodes, making up the majority of Depressive and Bipolar Disorders. In DSM-5, they are split up into Bipolar and Related Disorders and Depressive Mood Disorders.

Depression, elation, and irritability are cardinal signs in the primary disturbance of affect or mood. Abnormal affect or mood colours or exaggerates other mental functions.

Depressive Illness

In the updated "**2004** Global Burden of Disease Study **(WHO)**, depression was found to be the **third** leading cause of burden of disease **worldwide** and the **top** leading cause of burden of disease in **middle** and **high income countries**" (MOH Clinical Practice Guidelines 1/2012). However, there was no mention on the "cause" of depression.

The word **depression** can denote a **symptom, illness,** or **syndrome**. One can be depressed (i.e., feeling sad or low in spirit) but not suffering from a depressive illness. Depression as an illness is characterised by **low mood, psychomotor retardation or agitation**, and **negative beliefs**, also often with **loss of concentration** and **anhedonia** (i.e., loss of energy, interest, libido, and pleasure). For the newly initiated, it can be confusing to read about **melancholia, bipolar depression, "unipolar" depression** (i.e., without hypomania/mania), **major depressive disorder** (MDD; i.e., until occurrence of hypomania/mania), **psychotic depression** (with delusion and hallucination), **dysthymia** (which used to mean **neurotic** depression, later a **personality** disorder, and currently **chronic depressive mood disorder** that is long standing), and **"reactive" depression** (author's view). There are also special descriptions of **postpartum blues** and **depression in pueperium.** Prolonged and abnormal grief of bereavement exists now as a separate **prolonged grief disorder**. Thus, the **classification** of depression is not quite resolved. Besides, depression may be **primary, secondary**, or **organic.**

In recent years, with more new antidepressants available, it has been proclaimed that depression is widely prevalent and grossly **under-diagnosed** as well as **under-treated**. There is hardly any mention of why the malady has become so universally common. Most probably, more people are suffering from depression because of **increased stress** with **losses** associated with modern living, but this is not highlighted or is ignored. A consequence is the undesirable effects of focusing only on symptoms, overlooking causative factors, and encouraging medications. The medical principle of diagnosing and managing diseases according to aetiology appears to have been forgotten. For these sufferers, jobs creation and financial assistance during economic crises are probably more helpful in relieving stress and depression than medications.

Thus, the past **aetiological** concept of **endogenous** (inborn/ inherent or **genetic**) and **exogenous** (reactive or secondary) **depression** and the **clinical** picture of **psychotic** or **neurotic depression** merit review. In the former, family history is important, though the external cause may be covert. But in the latter, we are particularly obliged to look for causes (e.g., **stressors** and **losses**) in order to know the patients better and understand their environments, rather than merely following a checklist of symptoms or a criteria-set approach to diagnosing.

The "endogenous" depressive illness as in **manic-depressive psychosis** (MDP; now known as **bipolar disorder**) would be **bipolar depression** when the bipolar disorder is established. Otherwise, **MDD** is diagnosed until an episode of hypomania/ mania appears. In the past, "unipolar" depression (without hypomania/mania) would be diagnosed as part of **MDP** even before occurrence of hypomanic/manic episodes because its characteristics differ from reactive/secondary depression.

In other words, the current bipolar disorder is often a **retrospective** diagnosis waiting for the appearance of a hypomanic/ manic episode. **MDD** is therefore a heterogeneous group of mixed endogenous and exogenous depressive illnesses. The implications of differentiating endogenous (unipolar or bipolar of MDP) depression from exogenous (reactive or secondary) depression are in treatment (mood stabiliser or antidepressant or antipsychotic), understanding the course of the illness, and long-term prophylactic management. In endogenous depression, there seems to be an **absence** of obvious loss, but the "exogenous" is mainly reactive to **external stressors** (i.e., overt loss, whether material/non-material or physical/psychological) and will probably include most major depressive disorders. The clinical picture of "psychotic" (as in endogenous condition) or "neurotic" (as in exogenous condition) is still useful. Implied in "neurotic condition" is the presence of **personality traits** as an additional factor. The division of categories is of course not always clear cut and there is much overlapping which is to be expected. Hence, the dimensional aspect is debated.

Clinicians in the **past** distinguished endogenous depression from exogenous depression based on non-understandable onset, being out of touch with reality, diurnal variation of mood, early waking, psychomotor retardation or agitation, mood congruent hallucinations and delusions, non-reactive response, and high suicidal risk. On careful inquiry, some may even show brief hypomanic symptoms known as "manic defense" before onset of the depression. The symptoms are thought to be more biological and cyclical. No such distinction appears to be necessary or inquired nowadays. Spontaneous onset and remission may occur.

In clinical practice, many if not the majority of depression cases observed are **secondary** to other disabling disorders or diseases as well as **reactive** to psychosocial and socioeconomic factors, which are ignored or neglected. Such depression is usually diagnosed as a primary disorder or a comorbid condition. In "**double depression**", there is an acute reactive or secondary depression superimposed on a chronic or **primary** (endogenous) depression due to ongoing unresolved accumulated losses.

Pathophysiology as Pathogenesis

In simplistic pathophysiological terms, it may be postulated that endogenous (inborn or inherent) depression is due to monoamine deficiency in the brain. Exogenous depression is mediated mainly through the hypothalamus-pituitary-adrenal (HPA) axis in response to stressors or losses in life. The initial output of noradrenaline and cortisol is adaptive and beneficial in response to crisis. However, when high levels of noradrenaline and cortisol are prolonged and sustained, they become toxic and harmful to the body, resulting in cardiovascular, metabolic, and autoimmune disorders. Both the monoamine deficiency and HPA response can cause hippocampal atrophy leading to similar depressive symptoms.

It is perhaps due to the close linkage between the primary (endogenous) depression and secondary/reactive (exogenous) depression from chain reactions or "one thing leads to another" that current classifications have dispensed with aetiology. However, what is "endogenous" as in manic-depressive can also be viewed as a "predisposed vulnerability" to external precipitating stressors or losses. In exogenous depression, stressors or losses are directly aetiological. Diagnosis also depends on the stage of assessment along the longitudinal development of the illness (see relations between Anxiety and Depression).

Suggestion

Regardless of the current system of classification to follow officially, it would be useful to think about what is endogenous and exogenous in clinical management. A provisional "aetiological" classification may consist of **endogenous depression** (primary, "unipolar", or bipolar) when there are no obvious or significant losses or stressors and **exogenous depression** (reactive, secondary, or comorbid) when there are overt losses. Only then will we be less likely to miss out or overlook "causative" factors, whether predisposing, precipitating, or perpetuating, and manage them accordingly with inclusive protective factors instead of just treating symptoms or diagnosis of depression with drugs.

Bipolar Disorders (Manic Depressive Psychoses)

These **recurrent** affective/mood disorders (considered to be endogenous in origin and psychotic in nature in the past) are similar to schizophrenia in prevalence and early age of onset. They may present with depressive episodes alone (**unipolar**) or mania/hypomania with/without depressive episodes (**bipolar** or **manic-depressive psychosis** in the past). However, nowadays, bipolar affective disorders are subclassified into **I** (with mania) and **II** (with hypomania) with further specifiers and thus have become more complex. Genetics and family history as well as environmental factors play important roles. The episode may be single in a lifetime or more commonly manifest as multiple random episodes of depression and mania/hypomania throughout the lifetime. As manic or hypomanic episodes may emerge much later than depressive episodes, the diagnosis of bipolar disorder is often made **in retrospect** or much delayed. However, bipolar depression with prominent retardation can be diagnosed early before the appearance of mania or hypomania. During the course of illness, there is a tendency for each subsequent episode to become longer in duration and the remission period to become shorter. The illness eventually becomes chronic with all round deterioration of mental and physical health. Bipolar disorder is also believed to have higher suicide risk and shows cognitive deficits as well.

A recent hypothesis is that with each episode there is a chain of reactions in brain adaptation to the induced stress to maintain short-term stability (i.e., "**allostasis**"). The main hormonal mediators of the **stress response**, cortisol and adrenaline, have both protective and damaging effects on the body. Over time, due to wear and tear from chronic stress on the central nervous system and the body, there is a cumulative cost or "**allostatic load**" that leads to atrophy of nerve cells in the brain. In the long run, there is also damage of the **cardiovascular, metabolic,** and **immune systems**. The patient becomes less resilient and more vulnerable to medical comorbidity, early ageing, and cognitive impairment. In chronic stress, it is postulated that there is **brain rewiring** in the hippocampus, prefrontal cortex, and amygdala via neurotrophins. Among neurotrophins and their receptors, **brain-derived neuro-trophic factor (BDNF)** is thought to play a highly important role. It is involved in **neurogenesis**, neuronal survival, neuronal maturation, maturation of neural developmental pathways, and adult synaptic plasticity and dendritic growth and is essential to long-term memory. In chronic stress, trauma (abuses), and acute psychotic episodes, BDNF levels are decreased. **Second-generation antipsychotics** as well as **lithium** in treatment are thought to be protective or preventive of such stress-induced **structural remodeling** through stimulation of BDNF expression.

Manic Illness

The clinical picture of **hypomania or mania** (more severe) may be considered as the opposite of depressive illness. The mood is primarily **elated** (or **irritable**) and there is **increase in activity** but with little achievement. The patient is charged with energy, needs little sleep or rest, occupies himself with activities, gets distracted easily, and interferes with others. He is full of confidence, optimism, and may even have grandiose ideas, plans, and missions. He may spend unnecessarily and excessively or make irrational decisions in business transactions and run into financial trouble. He is disinhibited and talks loudly, fast, and too much, often with clang association. When the condition is mild, his gaiety can be infectious, but when the condition is severe, he is both irritating and irritable. He becomes excited, hyperactive, disruptive, and dysfunctional and may even exhibit hallucinations, delusions, and violent behaviour. There may also be amplification or exaggeration of what he is thinking or experiencing (e.g., crying at a sad thought or complaining of a physical discomfort). There is accentuation of personality traits and personal experience.

In **cyclothymia**, a virtually lifelong affliction, there is a persistent instability of mood involving numerous periods of mild depression and mild elation but not amounting to bipolar affective disorder or recurrent depressive disorder.

Relation Between Anxiety and Depression

Depression (mostly **reactive** or **exogenous** in nature) may be said to **begin with losses** of, for instance, loved ones and relationships, health and wealth, success and status, power and pride, or employment and livelihood and **result in losses** in sleep, appetite, libido, concentration, and capacity for work, pleasure, interest, energy, hope, meaning, and purpose in life. Risk of severe depression culminates in suicide.

Other symptoms distinguishing the more **endogenous** bipolar disorder or manic-depressive psychosis include diurnal variation of mood, guilt feelings, nonreactive response, suicidal thoughts or intent, nihilistic delusion, and mood-congruent auditory hallucinations. In severe affective/mood disorders, mood-incongruent delusions and hallucinations or even Schneider's first rank symptoms may be present (in current criteria). Bodily symptoms like aches and pains (somatization) are common and may be complained of as medical illness. Among **Asians** and **third-world populations**, losses, afflictions, and privations in life are **accepted** and **suffered** as one's **fate** and **destiny, ordained** perhaps by **gods** and **heavens** rather than "depression" as an illness. In fact, there may be hope of changing fortunes and a better next life. **Major Depressive Disorder** is **heterogeneous**, mostly **reactive** or **secondary**, and does not distinguish between what is exogenous or endogenous.

Nonetheless in depression there is **incapacity**. Depressed patients anticipate tasks and commitments with anxiety.

Anxiety may be considered the "**mother of psychopathology**". It is frequently a **precursor** or **trigger**, a **reinforcing** or **exacerbating** factor, and an **associated** or **secondary** symptom of many mental disorders. Hence, there is initial improvement when anti-anxiety drugs are prescribed for undifferentiated mental disorders at the primary care level.

How depressed and anxious the patient is depends on the **stage of development** and **time of presentation** of illness. It is not without reason that symptoms of **depression** and **anxiety** are frequently found together. When there is a "**loss**", be it **material** or **non-material**, or **physical** or **psychological**, depression will be experienced. In this state of depression, the individual will find tasks such as job assignments, life events, social activities, chores of daily living, and even festive celebrations **daunting** and **threatening**. He or she will also begin to experience anxiety or worry as these tasks are perceived as stressful. In this state of anxiety, he or she will not function optimally and suffer **loss in performance**, so in addition to anxiety, he or she will have depression. Anxiety is about what lies **ahead** while depression is about what has occurred **behind**.

Understanding of Stress and Chain Reaction

There is constant change in life due to relentless competition in the survival of the fittest.

When there is imposed change, there is a need to **adjust** and **adapt**.

External imposed changes without **control** and **choice** becomes a threat or stress.

The following simplified schemes may illustrate in **psychodynamic** terms the relationship between "**loss and depression**" and "**tasks and anxiety**":

(When there is pressure in life with loss of control and choice, stress will be experienced.)

Pressure ➔ Loss of Control and Choice ➔ Stress

When under stress and faced with tasks, anxiety will be experienced.

STRESS + TASK ➔ ANXIETY

When under stress with loss of capability or capacity, depression will be experienced.

STRESS + LOSS ➔ DEPRESSION

Loss leads to depression and when faced with tasks, anxiety is added.

LOSS ➔ DEPRESSION + TASK ➔ ANXIETY

Tasks lead to anxiety and when there is loss of capability or capacity, depression is added.

TASK ➔ ANXIETY + LOSS ➔ DEPRESSION

The proportion of anxiety and depression in **mixed anxiety-depression** depends on the stage of presentation between **tasks** and **losses.**

Development or Progression of Depression/Anxiety (Mixed States are more Common)

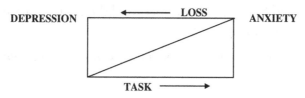

"Aetiology"

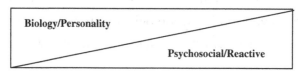

Clinical Presentation

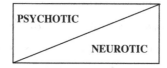

What do Suicides have in Common?

Edwin S. Schneidman, the Emeritus Professor of Thanatology at UCLA, draws up a list of "Ten Commonalities of Suicide". [Suicide (Guidelines for Assessment, Management & Treatment) Edited by Bruce Bongar, 1992] The list is as follows:

1. The common *purpose* of suicide is to seek a *solution*:
   Suicide is a problem-solving behaviour, not a random, pointless, or purposeless act

2. The common *goal* of suicide is *cessation of consciousness*:
    An urgently felt need to stop unbearable anguish; an action to
    put an end to intolerable affects and the individual's unwilling-
    ness to tolerate that pain

3. The common *stimulus* in suicide is *intolerable psychological
    pain*:
    Psychological pain is the centre of suicide and the basic clin-
    ical rule is to reduce the level of suffering, often just enough
    so that the individual can choose to live. In clinical practice,
    suicide prevention is psychological pain management.

4. The common *stressor* in suicide is *frustrated psychological
    needs*:
    It is a reaction to unfulfilled psychological needs. There are
    many pointless deaths but never a needless suicide. Frustrat-
    ed needs should be addressed.

5. The common *emotion* in suicide is *hopelessness-helplessness*:
    Feeling helpless and hopeless is pervasive in suicide.

6. The common *cognitive state* in suicide is *ambivalence*:
    Therapists use these simultaneous contradictory feelings to
    buy time.

7. The common *perceptual state* in suicide is *constriction*:
    There is a more or less transient psychological constriction of
    affect and intellect during which options are reduced to only
    one left.

8. The common *action* in suicide is *escape (egression)*:
    Egression is a person's intended departure from a region of
    distress.

9. The common *interpersonal act* in suicide is *communication of
    intention*:
    In most cases (80%), there were clear verbal or behavioural
    clues to the impending lethal event.

10. The common *consistency* in suicide is with *lifelong coping patterns*:
    We must look to previous episodes of deep perturbation, distress, duress, threat, and the capacity to endure psychological pain in order to find paradigms of egression in the suicidal person's life.

The high risk of suicide is seen as the climax reached in **pain** (psychological), **perturbation** (state of being upset or perturbed), and **press** (negative as opposed to positive conditions or events; e.g., good genes, happy fortune). The aim of management is to reduce pain, perturbation, and press that is negative. One should not confuse concomitance of events with causality of suicide. Clinically, a combination of depression and anxiety portends a high risk for suicide

"Neurotic" and Stress-Related Disorders

In **ICD-11, anxiety and fear-related disorders, obsessive-compulsive or related disorders, disorders specifically associated with stress, dissociative disorders,** and **disorders of bodily distress or body experience** are organised in separate blocks.

To understand changes in classification and nomenclatures, a brief review of the historical evolution in development may be in order.

The **Freudian** syndrome of **"anxiety neurosis"** includes symptoms of general irritability, chronic apprehension, or anxious expectation such as excessive worry, anxiety attacks (now called panic attacks), and secondary phobic avoidance. This "anxiety neurosis" was later renamed **"anxiety disorder"**. There were other "hysterical", "hypochondriacal", "neurasthenic", and "depressive neuroses" as well post-traumatic stress disorder and atypical anxiety disorder, which have been added to anxiety disorders. The earlier described anxiety neurosis with panic attacks became **generalised anxiety disorder**, an independent entity in DSM-III (1980) and in ICD-10 (1992), while the panic symptoms were separated into panic disorder. The "**phobic neurosis**" consists of agoraphobia with or without panic attack, social phobia, and simple phobia. Obsessive-impulsive neurosis has also been renamed obsessive-compulsive disorder.

Thus, **neuroses** or **neurotic disorders** are no longer mentioned as a class of mental disorders. Instead, specific disorders like anxiety, obsessive-compulsive, and somatic symptom and related disorders (DSM-5) are used. Nevertheless, the traditional concept and usage of "neurosis" remain popular. Neurotic symptoms are a result of interaction between the individual and his environment. By and large, **psychopathology** may be traced to past traumatic events, emotional conflicts, conditioning and learning of non-adaptive responses, and personality development from childhood to adulthood. All of these could be due to **exposure to** and **experience of** certain environments and upbringing that are **culturally determined** for the individual. The **symptomatology** is not always clear-cut for each case and is indeed often mixed. **Diagnosis** is made depending on whether emphasis is placed on the **dominant symptom** manifested, the **personality makeup** of the complainant, or the **environmental factors** prevailing. Different mental glossaries may describe differing categories of neurotic disorders based on symptoms, mental mechanisms, or reactions.

Aetiological Postulations

Much of mental life is believed to be **unconscious** in which are hidden the instinctual drives and forbidden desires seeking gratification. Also in the unconscious are forgotten memories accumulated from birth, whose attendant emotions still haunt and influence the individual through life. The conscious self normally copes by balancing the demands of instincts, reality, and the ideal. What are unacceptable, unpleasant, and painful are kept buried in the unconscious. In this way, **anxiety**, the primary and principal manifestation of emotional conflict, is prevented from troubling the mind. However, when the individual for some reason or other fails to maintain satisfactory mental equilibrium, anxiety emerges. Anxiety may be experienced either **directly** or **disguised** to appear as various physical or psychological conditions.

Thus, it has been hypothesised that unconscious anxiety may undergo complete conversion to physical or somatic symptoms, leaving the individual to feel "indifference" as in **hysteria or dissociation**. Or the anxiety may be focused on specific objects or situations as **phobias** that can be avoided. Or it can be **disguised** as rituals, a form of **magical undoing** in obsessive-compulsive disorders. When these mechanisms fail, the individual may experience free floating anxiety as in **generalised anxiety disorder (GAD)**.

The **behaviourist** believes that feelings and behaviours are a result of conditioning and learning (e.g., upbringing, parenting). People become neurotic when they either learn non-adaptive behaviour or fail to learn adaptive behaviour. **Biological proponents** talk of receptors in the brain, neurotransmitters, and genetic predisposition.

The experience of worry or anxiety, fear, nervousness, and tension is **universal**. When appropriate, it has survival value as it prepares the individual to protect himself from danger or threat; or enables him to compete and excel. There is also **existential** anxiety of life's inevitability or eventuality.

Generalised Anxiety Disorder

GAD is a new term for old anxiety neurosis with anxiety attacks but with shifting criteria and uncertain pathophysiology. To begin with, the panic attacks have been separated to go under panic disorder. In DSM-III to -IIIR and -IV, the duration criterion has been extended from 1 to 6 months and there is a shift of emphasis away from somatic complaints to psychological symptoms of "uncontrollable worry". ICD-10 is more practical, giving weight to both physical and psychological symptoms and a duration criterion of several months. Due to frequent symptoms of comorbidity especially associated with depression, it is debated whether GAD is an independent disorder or a trait or temperament vulnerability that overlaps with some depression. This has implications for management and the choice of treatment [see section on Affective (Mood) Disorders].

Phobic Anxiety Disorders

The common Phobic Anxiety Disorders include Agoraphobia with/without Panic disorder, Social Phobias, Specific (isolated), Phobias, and others.

Agoraphobia

The term means fear of open spaces. However, as a clinical entity, the fear includes public places, crowds, shops, cinemas, banks, and buses, especially when the patient is by himself. This eventually leads to the fear of leaving home, becoming house bound, and even being alone. The fear is related to the intense sense of insecurity that something may happen and the patient finds himself helpless or humiliated with no escape.

The development of agoraphobia is like the formation of a snowball. It may start with a dizzy spell or fainting attack in a public area. This may be followed by uneasiness of recurrence that gradually takes hold of the patient. He becomes sensitive to crowds and noises that over-arouse him and begins to develop both mental and physical symptoms of anxiety in such situations. Consequently, the person avoids these places. As time goes on, his fear is extended to cover more areas and his activities become more restricted. Eventually, he only feels safe at home. He can go out and travel a short distance only if accompanied, even by a child. The worst form is when he fears being alone even at home. It leads to **separation anxiety disorder**.

Social and Specific Phobias

Social phobias refer to **discrete situations** in which the patient fears that his appearance or actions are **under scrutiny** by other people. Symptoms of anxiety may develop when eating alone, speaking in public, or meeting the opposite sex at a social gathering. He therefore avoids such situations. These phobias usually start early in life and are associated with low self-esteem and fear of criticism.

Specific phobias refer to fear of animals, darkness, heights, enclosed spaces, flying, riding a lift, using public toilets, blood, disease, etc.

Panic Disorder

The symptoms that make up a **panic attack** occur in both medical disease and mental disorder. However, the diagnosis of the **panic disorder** (episodic paroxysmal anxiety) is described in ICD-10 as recurrent attacks of severe anxiety (panic) that are not restricted to any particular situation or set of circumstances and are **unpredictable. Dominant symptoms** vary from person to person, but sudden onset of palpitations, chest pain, choking sensations, dyspnoea, sweating, trembling, dizziness, and feelings of unreality (depersonalization or derealization) are common. There is **secondary fear** of dying, going mad, and losing control. The episode usually lasts minutes only but are sometimes longer. Frequency of attacks and its course are variable.

The panic attack itself is experienced as a **crescendo of fear** and **autonomic symptoms**, causing the person to make a hurried exit from the prevailing situation and subsequently engage in avoidance. Frequent and unpredictable panic attacks produce fear of being alone or going into public places. A panic attack is often followed by a persistent fear of having another attack.

Stages in development/progress of **Panic Disorder**

The following stages of panic disorder and how they progress and worsen when undiagnosed and untreated have been described by **David Sheehan** (USA):

Limited symptom attacks (i.e., fewer than four symptoms)

Panic attack → Health fears → Limited phobias → Extensive phobias → Depression.

Panic disorder is a **heterogeneous** group involving **different neurotransmitters**. Therefore, different drugs may be efficacious in its treatment.

Mixed Anxiety Disorders

Often, symptoms are mixed and not clear-cut enough to be given separate independent diagnoses. The commonest is **anxiety depression** (see relations between anxiety and depression). Others may include a mixture of obsessional and somatic symptoms.

Obsessive-Compulsive Disorder (OCD)

There is a wise **quote/saying** that is attributed to various sources:
"Beware of your **thoughts** for they become words.
Beware of your **words** for they become actions/deeds.
Beware of your **actions/deeds** for they become habits.
Beware of your **habits** for they become your character.
And your **character** becomes your **destiny**."

Obsessional trait involves preoccupation with **perfectionism**, resulting in **ambivalence**, constant **doubt**, and **indecision**. In life, some **optimal** level of obsessional trait is necessary for **success**.

Obsessive-compulsive disorder (OCD) in DSM-5 is grouped together with body dysmorphic disorder, hoarding disorder, trichotillomania, and excoriation disorder instead of under anxiety disorders. It can be a most distressing and incapacitating illness. OCD in ICD-11 is grouped likewise and includes hypochondriasis. The compulsive behaviour appears to be the common reason. Patients may have difficulty describing their symptoms as they may be affective, cognitive, or delusional and are sometimes misunderstood and thought to be psychotic. Leading questions may have to be asked to elicit diagnosis.

Clinical OCD

Consists of two components:

1. **Obsessive symptoms** — that which is said to be **anxiogenic** (i.e., causing anxiety) and includes **obsessive ruminations** of **involuntary** but **non-alien**, **intrusive**, and **recurrent thoughts** (cognitive), **images** (sensory), and **impulses/urges** (affective), often of an aggressive or obscene nature with fear of doing something harmful and wicked.

2. **Compulsive symptoms** — that which is said to be **anxiolytic**
   (i.e., relieving of anxiety) and includes both **repetitive physical rituals** (e.g., washing and checking) and ruminating **mental rituals** which may lead to compulsive action.

The individual recognises these symptoms as being **senseless**
and **unpleasant**. Efforts to **resist** them are unsuccessful because
of tension experienced. In the late stages of the illness, the individual may just give up resisting the compulsion. **OCD** may be associated with other mental disorders (e.g., schizophrenia, depression,
anxiety disorders) and there are sub-classifications specifying the
degree of insight into symptoms. The "**contents**" of obsessional
rumination are important and will be discussed later.

Compulsive acts and rituals are particularly represented in
the form of **repeated checking** and **washing**. The patient **feels
doubt** and checks his belongings, accounts, work, or more mundane things like the water tap, electric switch, gas oven, or doors
over and over again. If he is a "washer", he washes the things he
uses and himself to feel clean. For both checking and washing, he
may develop certain formulae and rituals to overcome excesses or
to feel satisfied. The secondary effect is that he develops fear of
dirt and excessive washing. He may then avoid washing altogether
and becomes filthy. He may also be compelled to read, count, walk,
touch, or behave certain ways to relieve inner tension. He can be
most trying by asking the same question repeatedly for reassurance.

The obsessive and compulsive components may be **separate**
and **independent** or **associated**. Their symptoms may undergo
endless **bizarre elaboration** or **substitution** as in **compulsive
mental rituals** before a simple action or task is carried out. The
sufferer is cognitively aware of his behaviour but feels compelled
to continue until he achieves "**satisfaction**". Normally, thinking,

acting, and feeling go hand in hand, but in this case, feeling lags behind knowing or there is "**affective lagging**".

Pathogenesis of OCD and Treatment

Research evidence (e.g., functional brain images) indicates that there is dysfunction in the complex cortico-striatal-thalamic-cortical neurocircuitry in OCD and other related compulsive and impulsive disorders. Lesions to basal ganglia causing OCD include **infections, immunologic causes, toxic substances, vascular infarction**, and **genetic** or **idiopathic** factors. **Post-encephalitic Parkinsonism** is known to exhibit OCD symptoms.

Serotonin deficiency is thought to play a major role in the production of OCD and other related impulsive and compulsive disorders, such as Gilles de la Tourette, trichotillomania, bulimia, and addictive behaviours. OCD symptoms may be induced by atypical antipsychotics (e.g., risperidone, clozapine) that are also $5HT_2$ antagonists. Dopamine and other neurotransmitters may also be involved. **Selective serotonin reuptake inhibitors** (SSRIs) and clomipramine (a tricyclic antidepressant) form the mainstay in pharmacotherapy of OCD. Recently, clinical reports suggest that **memantine**, an antagonist of NMDA receptors of the excitatory glutamate system, may be efficacious in OCD treatment.

Onset of OCD usually occurs in adolescence but consultation and diagnosis are often delayed until young adulthood. In terms of prognosis, only about **20%** will achieve full and sustained remission while **10%** become intractable and chronic. The rest shows **suboptimal** response to treatment. For intractable and chronic cases, irreversible **neurosurgery** might sometimes be considered. Strict ethical approval is required. The more recent **deep brain stimulation** is less drastic, but also requires the same approval. Behaviour therapy is also efficacious in normalising cortico-striatal-thalamic-cortical neurocircuitry dysfunction and is preferred as a first-line treatment for younger patients. Combination of psychopharmacotherapy and behaviour therapy may produce better results.

An empirical postulation based on anecdotal experience

It is postulated that **obsessive rumination** may be "**conscious**" and present as **OCD** symptoms or "**unconscious**" and manifest as **auditory hallucinations** and **delusional ideas** like in **schizophrenia**. "**Obsessive rumination**" in the **unconscious mind** is akin to many applications running simultaneously in the background of a computer that **pop up** (as advertisements or reminders) on the screen, just like psychotic symptoms. Long-term sufferers may reveal insight on the source of their symptoms.

As mentioned earlier, "**contents**" of obsessive rumination (conscious and unconscious) can explain the occurrence of both OCD and many other anxiety or mental disorders.

Mental disorders in individuals with **obsessive ruminations** may include:

Phobia — when **content** is about phobic objects and situations such as dirt, disease, and death

Post-Traumatic Stress Disorder — when **content** is about past experiences, trauma, and memories

Anorexia Nervosa — when **content** is about weight and obesity

Hypochondriasis — when **content** is about physical or mental symptoms with no known causes

Dysmorphophobia — when **content** is about preoccupation with bodily appearance

Schizophrenia — when **content** is more likely **unconscious** but emerging into consciousness as auditory hallucinations and delusional ideas

Insomnia — when a patient is kept awake due to obsessive rumination before sleep

Kleptomania — a controversial mental disorder in **forensic** practice illustrating components of situational obsessive impulses or urges that are anxiogenic and lead to compulsive commission of offences that are anxiolytic.

Other conditions such as **autism** and **early stages of addictive behaviour** might be similarly affected.

Experience-based observation:
Up to half of some 40 **anecdotal** cases handled by the author with the abovementioned postulated psychopathology have shown improvement with adjunct SSRIs and zolpidem treatment. Incidentally, zolpidem is a hypnotic and anxiolytic but may also have anti-obsessional actions or properties.

Research needs to be done to confirm or support these clinical observation.

Other Stress-Related Disorders

In **Acute Stress Reaction, Adjustment Disorder**, and **Post-Traumatic Stress Disorder**, the focus is on the **precipitating stressor** or **aetiology**. The **symptomatology** is **variable** depending on the vulnerability of the individual and severity of the circumstance. Symptoms may range from **neurotic** to **psychotic** (e.g., anxiety, depression, conversion symptoms, dissociative phenomena, hallucinations, delusions) and be diagnosed as **syndromes**.

Post-Traumatic Stress Disorder (PTSD) first appeared in DSM III (1980) and ICD-10 (1992). It had existed in the past as "shell shock", "battle fatigue", "trauma neurosis", and in some cases "compensation neurosis". However, its aetiological criteria in the DSM have evolved from exceptional trauma that would affect almost anyone to milder traumatic events such as accidents and assault. Furthermore, one can also be affected by witnessing such events being experienced by others. Finally, such events so defined include acute reactions involving intense fear, helplessness, or horror. In other words, the focus is shifted to the individual's reactions rather than on the aetiological event. ICD-10 has kept to the initial definition of PTSD that it arises as a delayed and/or protracted response to an exceptionally stressful event or situation, such as a natural disaster or human violence that would affect almost anyone. Symptoms of Acute Stress Reaction, such as initial daze or numbness, intense mixed emotions (e.g., fear, despair, anger, depersonalization), and withdrawal or overactivity which occur immediately or within minutes of the trauma instead of resolving within few days, can persist up to 3–6 months. In addition, there are "**flashbacks**" or persistent **re-experience** of the traumatic stressor in the form of **recurrent intrusive recollections, recurrent distressing dreams**, and **reliving of the traumatic event**. Victims also show **avoidance** (including dissociative symptoms) of anything associated with the traumatic event and **increased arousal state** or excitability. Symptoms of anxiety and depression are common. There may be delayed onset of symptoms up to six months after the traumatic event.

In **ICD-11**, the definition of **PTSD** includes the above; that is, (1) re-experiencing the traumatic event(s) in the form of vivid intrusive memories, flashbacks, or nightmares accompanied by overwhelming emotions of fear or horror as well as intense physical sensations; (2) avoidance of associated thoughts, memories, activities, situations, or people reminiscent of the event(s); (3) persistent perceptions of current heightened threat such as startling reactions to unexpected noises. The symptoms must persist for at least several weeks and cause significant impairment in personal, family, social, educational, occupational, or other important areas of functioning.

Over the years, the concept of PTSD has undergone changes and is being debated. The latest research regards the pathophysiology of PTSD as an **attachment disorder** (i.e., insecure attachments) and the most important **risk factor** is **lack of social support**. The **right** cerebral hemisphere, hypothalamic pituitary adrenal (**HPA**) system, and **hippocampus** are believed to be involved. Thus, cognitive and verbal therapy involving mainly the left hemisphere is inadequate. Unlike other stress reactions, the corticotrophin-releasing factor is raised but the cortisol level is low.

Sleep Disorders

Sleep is very important for both physical and mental health. During sleep, the body repairs itself after the day's physical wear and tear and the mind restores itself to maintain optimal functioning. Sleep is therefore necessary as well as therapeutic when one is ill. However, the quantity and quality of sleep are believed to decline gradually after adulthood. There is less deep and more interrupted sleep.

The **staging** and **phasing** of sleep, like all biological data, shows normal variation. **Normal sleep** may be divided into two kinds — non-rapid eye movement sleep (i.e., **non-REM** or quiet sleep) and rapid eye movement sleep [i.e., **REM** (active or paradoxical) sleep]. They go in cycles from **Stage 1** which is transitional between wakefulness and sleep; **Stage 2** which involves light sleep; **Stage 3** which is transitional between light and deep sleep; to **Stage 4** which is REM sleep.

Deep sleep occurs in the **non-REM** phase which is supposed to be free from dreams. The vital signs are regular and stable, reflecting a resting state, and it is physically restorative. However, muscle tone is present and the individual is capable of movement. In **REM sleep**, dreams occur and there is scanning movement of the eyes. The vital signs are "activated" and irregular and there is penile tumescence in the male. However, voluntary muscles are in a flaccid state and the individual seems paralysed. Thus, in **somnambulism** and **night terror** that occur in deep sleep, the individual is capable of physical movement but has no recall. On the other hand, in **nightmares**, the individual experiences frightening dreams but feels paralysed and trapped. Diazepam, which lightens deep sleep, helps in somnambulism, night terror, and bed wetting.

Sleep disorders may be primary or secondary. Common primary sleep disorders include obstructive sleep apnoea (**OSA**) and periodic limb movement disorder (**PLMD**) due to endogenous disturbances. Diagnostic evaluation can be carried out using polysomnography (**PSG**). Secondary sleep disorders covers a host of medical, psychological, and environmental factors such as arthritis, depression, and disturbing surroundings.

A sleep disorder of special interest is **Narcolepsy**, which is characterised by the tetrad of excessive daytime sleepiness, cataplexy, hypnagogic/hynopompic hallucination, and sleep paralysis. Not all four are always present in every patient. In cataplexy, there is sudden loss of muscle tone brought on by strong emotions (e.g., "buckling of knees from laughter") or falling. Patients may also complain of fatigue, low mood, obesity, clumsiness, slurring speech, falling asleep during activity, and poor performance. Daytime naps may be restorative. Narcolepsy is a neurological disturbance, but the current understanding is that it is an **autoimmune disorder** following an

infection or **injury** and is more common in adolescents. Low CSF **hypocretin** measurement is diagnostic. Hypocretin neurons in the hypothalamus are involved in stimulating other brain cells to facilitate staying awake. Treatment of narcolepsy includes psychostimulants and specific antidepressants. Off-label use of sodium oxybate ameliorates cataplexy. In **delayed sleep phase disorder**, there is late onset of sleep and delay in waking up. Sometimes, the parameters in non-REM and REM sleep seem to have become "disrupted" or "dissociated" and one gets mixed kinds of sleep disorders.

As one grows older, sleep becomes intermittent and there is reduction of deep sleep and duration of sleep. Sleep apnoea (interruption of breathing during sleep) from organic causes is increasingly diagnosed and treated nowadays.

Dreams are brain activities during sleep in the **REM** phase. There have been psychoanalytical explanations and interpretations of their function and significance. Physiologically, the physical body is repaired and mental capacity is restored during sleep. It is akin to the **defragmentation** process of the computer, which organises and assembles haphazardly saved data during waking to optimise working memory capacity and allow for more input. It is also analogous to the activities that go on in a **bank** or **library** after closing. Staff members stay back to sort out, classify, catalogue, and file the accounts, transactions, or returned books so that they can be ready for business again the next day. In the process of sorting and filing, they may come into contact with other adjacent accounts, files, or books, so we dream of not only what took place during the day but also related matters in the past. The materials may undergo editing or synthesising, perhaps in story form. In sleep deprivation, the materials of daily experiences and transactions are left unsorted and working memory capacity can be affected and mental functions disorganised. Sleep is therefore essential and therapeutic to mental and physical health. There is also "active dreaming" in "awareness". The content is like thought disorder in consciousness.

Culture-Bound Syndromes

These are **syndromal symptoms** and **behaviours** that **incorporate cultural beliefs** and **ideas** in **their causes** and **effects**. "**Koro**" is an example in which there is a perception of penile retraction into the body, a belief that it brings death and is accompanied by panic anxiety symptoms. Both sporadic and epidemic koro cases have occurred in Asia. Symptomatic koro that is secondary to schizophrenic delusion has also been reported.

Man has an innate desire to master and dominate his environment, which is evident in the human quest for knowledge, seeking explanations for observed phenomena, and deriving answers to problems. When faced with uncertainty or the unknown, he feels uneasy and threatened. A natural tendency is to ascribe to the supernatural what is inexplicable and unpredictable. In this way, it becomes easier to accept and communicate the distress or misfortune. Resignation to what is beyond control removes shame and stigma and makes life bearable.

As a general rule, people consult their family doctor for their physical ailments, the religious clergy for their spiritual troubles, and the psychiatrist for their emotional or mental symptoms. Thus, the religious clergy and the psychiatrist may see different groups of people in need of help. Each may describe the same phenomenon in his or her own language and terminology with apparent differences in opinion. Some prefer to call **trance states** and **spirit possessions** social diagnoses and therefore regard them as outside the field of medicine. Thus, depending on the operational definitions used, the same condition may be fixed with a **medical, sociocultural**, or **spiritual label**. From a medical point of view, nothing is more rewarding than to see a person recover from his affliction through proper interventions.

Trance states and **spirit possessions** are **dissociative phenomena**. According to William Sargent, the dissociation of consciousness in trance states is more or less complete and the individual's personality is temporarily displaced and taken over by someone else (e.g., a deity or spirit). Upon recovery, there is amnesia of what had taken place. In spirit possession, the individual is conscious of being possessed by some spirit that is in control of him. Culturally speaking, these phenomena serve certain personal and social functions. The belief in the discernment and pronouncement of the deity or spirit is a powerful influence in the therapeutic process. The deity or spirit at times enables the "weak" to speak their mind to the "strong" without fear of repercussion, and the "strong" are more prepared to listen to the deity or spirit speaking through the "weak" without loss of face. In this way, an intolerable situation might be resolved. It should not be dismissed as simply superstition.

However, there are unscrupulous mediums who make use of such belief in deities and spirits to deceive and cheat others who may be gullible, naïve, or under stress.

Eating disorders (i.e., **anorexia nervosa** and **bulimia nervosa**) may also be considered as a western culture-bound syndrome. The pursuit of thinness is a modern form of "glamour culture". In anorexia nervosa, there is not only a deliberate reduction of calorie intake but also increased effort in calorie expenditure. The belief is that one is too fat even when grossly underweight. In the related bulimia nervosa, there is bingeing of food followed by self-induced vomiting and purging to control weight. Interacting sociocultural (e.g., diet and eating habit) and biological (e.g., genetic and pubertal development) factors are probably involved in their psychopathology. However, many are believed to have underlying depression and low self-esteem or a strong need to be in control. In view of the seriousness of physical stigmata, endocrine abnormality, metabolic disturbance, and the real risk of mortality, management should be intensive, comprehensive, and sustained. A new periodic **bingeing disorder** has been added in DSM-5.

The symptoms may also be secondary to other mental disorders. Anxious patients may eat excessively to relieve anxiety or throw up because of anxiety. Depressed patients generally have poor appetites, but some may binge drink and eat. Schizophrenic patients may resist eating due to hallucinatory commands not to eat or delusional beliefs that their food has been poisoned. Management depends on the psychopathology.

Classic culture-bound syndromes such as **Koro, Latah**, and **Amok** seem to have disappeared from our region. What could be the explanation? Are culture-bound syndromes dependent on the prevailing cultural milieu or the society's stage of development? Some are of the opinion that when a society becomes more developed with advanced knowledge, the so-called culture-bound syndromes would disappear. The belief seems to be that all mental disorders can be reduced to common, biological, generic psychopathology and mechanisms (i.e., anxiety disorders, affective disorders, and psychoses). However, it may also be a matter of definition and nomenclature. For instance, to DSM users, neurasthenia is a form of depression whereas to the Chinese, it is an entity that may include depression.

Evolution and Hierarchy of Aetiological Concepts of Diseases

In the history of medicine, cause of disease has been attributed to the following factors:

Supernatural/Superstitious → Physical/Environmental → Biological/Organic/Genetic → Psychological/Social → Moral/Spiritual?

Within each culture and society, there are different evolutionary and hierarchical approaches to understanding illnesses or illness behaviours and their management. Much depends on the prevailing belief system and theoretical model, which may shape the manifestation and presentation of the disorder. Different healers or therapists are consulted.

5 Treatment and Management

Pharmacotherapy and Psychotherapy

The **brain** and **mind** dichotomy seems to be reflected in the proponents of **physical** and **psychological** methods of treatment. The psychopharmacological approach to treatment is to restore normal neurotransmission affected by "synaptopathy" or "defective connectivity". The rationale is to augment what is deficient and dampen what is excessive through the use of drugs that are agonists or antagonists in the systems concerned.

In simplistic terms, there are also the **GABA inhibitory system** and the **glutamate excitatory system**. They need to be in **optimal balance** for mental health. To achieve an inhibitory state, relevant or specific agonists of the GABA-ergic system, relevant or specific antagonists of the glutamatergic system, or both can be employed. Similarly, to achieve an excitatory state, antagonists of the GABA-ergic system, agonists of the glutamatergic system, or both can be employed. Polypharmacy may therefore be fine-tuned and enhanced for desired outcomes.

Lately, studies suggest that **antipsychotics** and **antidepressants or mood stabilisers** do not just act neurochemically as agonists or antagonists but can **stimulate** the **brain-derived**

neurotrophic factor (BDNF) to create new neural pathways. It is postulated that brain cells are damaged by illness and stress and BDNF promotes **neurogenesis** and **neuroplasticity**. In neurogenesis, existing nerve stem cells can differentiate into specific nerve cells. In neuroplasticity or brain or cortical plasticity, neurons exposed to normal experience or injury can undergo growth, reorganization, migration, and rewiring and assume new function.

Psychological treatment embraces, at one end, classical psychoanalytical psychotherapy and, at the other end, cognitive and behaviour therapy. Theories abound as to how symptoms are derived and how they can be relieved. Be it a therapeutic relationship or counselling, reconditioning or desensitization, meditation or mindfulness, hypnotic suggestion, abreaction, diversional therapy, cognitive change, positive stroke, or placebo response, the **mechanism** is intended to effect a **change** in the morbid pattern of neuronal circuitry. Morbid circuits may also be disrupted by aversion therapy, which is achieved through **strategic** and **systematic verbal**, **behavioural**, or **experiential input** to **re-channel** or **bypass** "prevailing faulty circuits" or **open or create** "new desirable circuits". It is likened to **rewiring**. **Effort** and **practice** (like **compliance or adherence** with medications) are necessary to maintain new pathways and improvements. The most powerful force to effect change is the arousal of **emotions** and "**love**". Happy memories or painful experiences are equally important in therapeutic processes.

Therefore, if the objective of **psychopharmacotherapy** is to restore normal neurotransmission, then the role of **psychotherapy** is to facilitate the direction of desirable neurotransmission. On the other hand, physical exercise, relaxation activities, meditation, and enjoyable diversions or hobbies provide breaks for overheated circuits to recover from excessive stress and cool down.

Physical exercise and **skill training** are thought to promote structural regeneration of cells in the hippocampus and their function. They also stimulate and integrate cognitive, affective, sensory, and motor functions.

It is also important to remember that neither is the mind of a psychotic person necessarily completely deranged nor is he psychotic all the time. There will always be a part of him that can function and respond normally. With patience and understanding, one can relate to this normal part of the mind and strengthen and expand it. This may explain the success of **charismatic therapists** because of **positive therapeutic relationships.**

Evidence-Based Medicine (EBM) and Treatment Algorithm

Nowadays, there is much emphasis or cliche on "**evidence-based medicine**", which derives from **clinical studies** that are **deductive**, while "**experience-based medicine**", which derives from **anecdotal insights** that are **inductive**, is neglected. In fact, evidence-based medicine **begins** with anecdotal observations and empirical experience. To insist rhetorically on "evidence" first before initiating any new and potentially beneficial treatment is to think within the box and impede innovation and progress. There would have been no discovery of the antibiotic penicillin and vaccination of chicken pox. Much depends on the **availability of facilities** and **resources to conduct research** so that experience-based becomes evidence-based.

In research, it is important to be mindful that the larger the samples and the longer the periods of studies, the simpler the statistics and the greater the validity and reliability of the findings will be. Conversely, the smaller the samples and the shorter the durations of clinical trials, the more complex the statistics and the lesser the validity and reliability of the results will be. That said, universal truth can be derived from studies of single cases while what is statistically correct may have no predictive value for individual cases.

In the management of psychiatric disorders as well as in general medicine and other specialties, **treatment algorithms** or guidelines in treatment are developed and taught. In psychiatry, such evidence-based medicine derives mainly from **randomised controlled drug trials** (RCTs), which are carried out on diagnostic categories dominated by DSM's definitions and criteria, standard questionnaires, or rating scales on symptoms, limited patient populations, fixed periods of time, and complex statistical analyses.

When there is inconsistency in published findings from different clinical drug trials, a **meta-analysis** (which excludes unpublished negative reports) is conducted. Strangely, in such clinical drug trials, the **response rates** of common mental disorders such as anxiety, depression, and schizophrenia, respectively, to each drug within the specific psychotropic class of anti-anxiety, antidepressant, and antipsychotic investigated have been **overall** about **1/3** to **2/3** (not excluding **placebo**) response.

The standard conclusion is that within each class of drugs, the **efficacy** for each disorder is about the **same** (i.e., antipsychotic A is as effective as antipsychotic B in the treatment of schizophrenia and antidepressant X is as effective as antidepressant Y in the treatment of major depression, and so on and so forth). The main difference or selling point is in the **side effect profile**, **adverse reaction**, or **specific domain investigated**. Clinical trials and treatments are **diagnoses-based**, which are heterogeneous and lack specificity. Typically, psychosocial factors are ignored and a holistic approach is neglected.

It is often asked by pharmaceutical presenters with vested interests whether all antipsychotics, antidepressants, anxiolytics, mood stabilisers, or anticonvulsants are the same, implying that some are superior to others. It might as well be asked whether all psychotic, bipolar, depressed, and anxious patients are the same. Patients may have the same diagnosis but respond differently to the same drug and in fact sometimes exhibit paradoxical reactions (e.g., activation instead of sedation). They also have **different psychosocial backgrounds** and **life events**.

Over the years, despite the up to two thirds response phenomenon, diagnostic categories have increased and become **more** differentiated, perhaps taking into account multi-factorial causes, varied manifestations, and courses (e.g., in affective and anxiety disorders). This might suggest more specific **nosological** entities being defined. However, in practice, psychopharmacotherapy has become **less** differentiated. Drugs **registered** originally for **specific** mental disorders are now promoted to treat, **off label**, other categories of mental disorders that may have **similar or shared common symptoms** or **psychopathology**, such as hallucinations, delusions, disturbed behaviour, or mood and suicidal risk as in schizophrenia, affective disorders, and organic brain syndromes. This is not surprising when the **drugs used do not actually act specifically on so-called specific disorders** but ameliorate overlapping symptoms in different disorders. The **crossing over** of drug treatment is also likely to be driven by expiry of the **patent** for a specific disorder and **market forces**. It is therefore necessary to carefully review the diagnosis of mental disorder, clinical drug trial, and the so-called evidence-based medicine in management. Furthermore, it makes sense to treat underlying **psychopathology** and/or **pathophysiology** as understood or postulated rather than as specific diagnosis without nosological basis or by consensus of opinion. There should be a **shift of paradigm** to focus on psychopathology and pathophysiology rather than operationalised diagnosis when conducting clinical drug trials.

More often than not, clinicians are guided in their prescriptions by their practical experience, knowledge, and understanding of psychopathology, pathophysiology, and individual psychosocial stressors of each patient besides factors such as availability, affordability, and lifestyle. Such individualised management will likely give better results than **one size fits all, trial and error algorithms of recommended drugs**.

Disparity in diagnosis and management among clinicians is therefore not surprising. Inadvertently, the so-called "off label" dynamic of polypharmacy creeps in. **RCTs** should therefore preferably be based on **psychopathology** and **pathophysiology** rather than on "specific" diagnosis. After all, we do **not** talk of "**anti-schizophrenic**" or "**anti-bipolar**" drugs even when RCTs are based on diagnoses of schizophrenia and bipolar disorder. We prescribe instead common **antipsychotics** or **mood stabilisers**.

As a matter of fact, due to overlapping of syndromes and multiple disorders diagnosed, drug treatment becomes undifferentiated and unspecific. There is already a trend to shift the focus on management of **specific domains** of psychopathology, such as functional cognitive deficits in **depressive illness** (as in the new antidepressant **vortioxetine**), to different domains of symptoms. It involves parameters of social function, work capacity, and productivity apart from sleep, mood, and libido. Likewise, specific domains of psychopathology in schizophrenia may respond to different antipsychotics.

Biomarkers are questionable when diagnoses are syndromal, non-nosological, and heterogeneous with shared genes and similar symptomatology. Besides, biomarkers can be either the "cause" or "effect". However, biomarkers are being looked into in terms of treatment response.

In general, the practice of evidence-based medicine is controlled by the FDA, other international academic or professional bodies, and individual national regulations. What is approved and available in one country may not be the same in another. They are not binding, comprehensive, and infallible. In fact, they may impede discovery and progress from experience-based observations.

Psychotherapy

Pharmacotherapy has come to a sort of "dead end" in recent years, with most patented drugs becoming generic and with very limited new drugs with novel mechanisms on the horizon. Ironically, efficacious generic drugs are not produced because of non-profitability. It is not surprising that psychotherapy is swinging back because RCTs have omitted psychosocial factors, whether intrapsychic or interpersonal in mental disorders, which are important in understanding morbidity and management. However, there are many schools, theories, and models on psychopathology and therefore a wide variety of psychotherapies. Psychotherapy probably works through plastic rewiring of neurocircuitries through systematic and strategic cognitive and behavioural input, while pharmacotherapy attempts to restore balance of neurotransmitters and synaptic receptors.

Community and Social Psychiatry are also growing in importance to provide comprehensive and holistic management.

The **guidelines** of the **World Federation of Societies of Biological Psychiatry (WFSBP)** are broadly as follows:

In the treatment of **schizophrenia**, the so-called atypical or second-generation antipsychotics have become the standard first choice. It seems to indicate that despite the higher cost and possible life-threatening side effects of metabolic disturbance in the form of obesity, diabetes mellitus, hyperlipidaemia, and cardiovascular complications that incur additional monitoring, treatment, and burden, these drugs are still preferred to conventional antipsychotics that induce non-life-threatening extra-pyramidal symptoms (EPS), **tardive dyskinesia** (TD), and perhaps negative symptoms.

For **bipolar mood (affective) disorders**, in particular **manic** or **hypo-manic** episodes (and subsequent maintenance), lithium is the treatment of choice and mood stabilisers, anticonvulsants, or antipsychotics can be used in monotherapy or in combination. For bipolar **depression**, sodium valproate, mood stabilisers, antipsychotics, and/or antidepressants are indicated. Antidepressants are mainly prescribed for depressive symptoms and should be tailed off when the depressive episode is over. There is controversy on the efficacy of antidepressants on bipolar depression in both therapy and prophylaxis as well as possible harm in causing acute mania and new **rapid cycling disorder** or cycle acceleration. Sodium valproate, mood stabilisers, or antipsychotics are preferred. Indeed, one should also be guided by one's own experience and the patient's response.

In the treatment of **anxiety spectrum disorders**, the different SSRIs have become the recommended first-line drugs. The benzodiazepines are more or less sidelined into secondary roles probably due to potential misuse and abuse or dependency and addiction. It is an overreaction to discourage or prohibit benzodiazepines. Psychotherapies such as cognitive behaviour therapy have been suggested to offer more sustainable long-term benefits. The general principle is that pharmacotherapy and psychotherapy combined produces better results.

Guidelines aside, **anxiety** may be considered the "**mother of psychopathology**" and is frequently a **precursor** or **trigger**, **reinforcing** or **exacerbating factor**, and **associated** or **secondary symptom** of many mental disorders. Thus, anti-anxiety drugs (whether SSRIs or benzodiazepine) are often useful in ameliorating most mental disorders and therefore widely prescribed at the primary healthcare level. **Polypharmacy**, though **not** to be encouraged, is hence unavoidable when symptoms are **dynamic** and **polymorphic**.

In psychiatry, the patient is not a diagnosis of symptoms. Moreover, the symptom checklist approach may miss underlying primary disorders and leave them untreated. It cannot be overemphasised that unless a thorough **biopsychosocial** assessment is conducted, **it is not uncommon that an inaccurate diagnosis is made, incorrect treatment is given, the patient neither improves nor dies, he does not complain, and we are none the wiser.** There is no place for smugness.

Management of Inpatients

Psychiatric management is multidisciplinary
Sleep is almost always affected during the acute stage of any mental condition. It is therefore therapeutic to ensure sleep and restore normal sleep patterns. The newly admitted patient, being in a strange environment, should be given adequate hypnotic or sedative medication Exceptions will be those who are semi-comatose or confused from organic causes (sodium amylobarbitone 200 mg to be taken at night had been most effective and useful, but unfortunately it is no more available). **Diazepam** 10 mg or **hydroxyzine** 25 mg at night are usually prescribed in our practice. There is actually a wide selection of **benzodiazepines** from **short**

to **long acting** to choose from, such as **lorazepam**, **midazolam**, and **flurazepam**. For the **depressed**, one of the more sedative antidepressants including **amitriptyline**, **trimipramine**, or **dothiepin** 25–50 mg or **mirtazapine** 15 mg may be prescribed. In the case of the **psychotic**, antipsychotic drugs like **chlorpromazine** or **thioridazine** (unfortunately out of production) 50–100 mg will promote sleep as well. Nowadays, **olanzapine** 5–10 mg and **quetiapine** 25–50 mg are more often prescribed. For those with disturbed **organic** conditions with clouding of consciousness, **haloperidol** 1.5–5 mg may be helpful (see treatment of insomnia).

Acutely **disturbed** and **violent** patients should be sedated and restrained when necessary. Oral antipsychotics (e.g., clozapine 25–50 mg) and benzodiazepines (e.g., lorazepam 1mg) may be given, short term, in close intervals if the patient can be persuaded. Otherwise, i/m haloperidol 5–10 mg for the psychotic is preferred, although i/m chlorpromazine 50–100 mg can be given too. The latter may cause postural hypotension and falls (i/m paraldehyde is not an antipsychotic but a powerful and quick sedative that is no longer in use). For maintenance of sedation, medication can be repeated as and when necessary either orally or by injection. Injection of **clopixol acuphase** 50–100 mg is useful in providing sedation for up to 24–48 hours (e.g., over the weekend). Others may prefer midazolam injection. Some may object to sedative "drugging". Difficult and unstable patients may be referred to the High Dependency Unit for management.

In restraining the patient, proper procedures and regular monitoring of vital signs should be observed. When sedation has taken effect, restraints should be released. The patient may be "isolated" separately and other patients should be kept away.

All new admissions should be reviewed by an Associate Consultant/Consultant. Ideally, a **multidisciplinary team** consisting of psychiatrists or doctors, nurses, medical social workers, clinical psychologists, occupational therapists, case managers, and pharmacists should see the case together for total management.

The mental state of organic cases with confusion should be reviewed **daily** for **orientation, memory,** and **vital signs.** A neurological examination should be performed. Often, they are referred directly to general hospitals to assess for and exclude brain lesions.

Patients who are **recurrently** disturbed and violent should be carefully reviewed with the aim of understanding the nature of his behaviour. Often, reports of such behaviour result in escalation of medication. A more fruitful approach is to determine whether the behaviour is in **response to psychotic experience; impulsive, compulsive, or hyperactive in nature; due to epilepsy or akathisia;** and so on. Treatment can then be more rationalised and tailored according to clinical formulations.

TREATMENT — Physical, Psychological, Social

A. Physical Treatment

Physical treatment includes **pharmacotherapy, electroconvulsive therapy** (ECT), and more recently **transcranial magnetic stimulation** (TMS). **Brain surgery** or **psychosurgery** and **deep brain stimulation** are not done here. Pharmacotherapy is, of course, the mainstay.

Pharmacotherapy

Psychotropic drugs include the **anti-anxiety** (anxiolytic or minor tranquilliser), **antidepressant, anti-manic, antipsychotic** (major tranquilliser), **mood stabilisers,** and others. Within each category, there are numerous choices available. **Statistically,** the efficacy of the different drugs in each category is about equal and the selling point is in the different side effect profiles claimed. In most drug trials, the **overall response rate** of **each drug** is from **one third** to **two thirds** including placebo effects. However, we are not told which **two thirds** would respond to which drug. One possible explanation is that psychiatric disorder and treatment is **not** well differentiated and specific enough. The pathophysiology or mechanisms are not fully understood and psychosocial factors are not considered. Although polypharmacy is discouraged, it is in fact fairly prevalent in practice and not without rationale. For instance, a less sedative drug can be prescribed during the day and a more sedative drug at night. A **combination of drugs** may improve symptoms more than the prescription of a single drug as the efficacy of each drug, although similar (i.e., up to two thirds), does not overlap completely. Effects may also be due to drug interaction.

Psychiatric treatment or psychopharmacotherapy is **symptomatic** and thus no different from the management of chronic arthritic, asthmatic, diabetic, epileptic, hypertensive, and a host of other cardiac, dermatological, immunological, and neurological conditions, which is also not curative. So far, research and clinical trials focus primarily on symptoms reduction as evidence of effectiveness. However, absence of symptoms does not mean being capable of functioning and presence of symptoms does not preclude reasonable functioning. Recovery of functions is now emphasised. Psychosocial factors, stressors, and cultural and environmental influences are frequently ignored.

More recently, there has been a shift toward **subjective indices** such as patient's self-reports on **quality of life**. Apart from objective research findings and subjective reports of satisfaction, a third possible area for inquiry could be the **carer's or family's**

views on the therapeutic outcome. A complete biopsychosocial assessment of each patient is therefore necessary. Besides drugs, **holistic milieu therapy** is just as important. However, **covert** treatment or medication is disallowed or discouraged ethically. The reason is that individual rights are sacrosanct. However, such absolute rights can be dubious when they affect other people's rights to safety, wellbeing, and peace of mind.

Early diagnosis and treatment cannot be overemphasised because of chain reactions and the cumulative deleterious effects of illness. However, it must be kept in mind that all drugs may have side or adverse effects. In clinical practice, we diagnose and treat according to aetiology or rather **pathophysiology**. For instance, in cases of myocardial infarction or stroke, we do not just treat the diagnosis per se in terms of thrombosis or haemorrhage but also the attendant hypertension, hyperlipidaemia, diabetes mellitus, and other contributing causes. As the trend towards **polypharmacy** is unavoidable, attention should be paid to **drug–drug interactions**. The liver **cytochrome P450** enzymes system metabolises different drugs at different rates and to different extents. Due to **individual** and **ethnic** differences, the therapeutic dosage of each drug must be varied or adjusted. When drugs are used in combination, there is an additional consideration of metabolic competition between drugs and enzymes. As a result, the **efficacy** or **toxicity** of each drug used in combination with other drugs may be affected.

The **principles** of symptomatic treatment are as follows:

1. <u>Therapeutic Phase</u>

Some clinicians prefer to start with larger doses for quick efficacy and titrate downwards to reduce side effects, whereas others prefer to start with smaller doses to avoid side effects and titrate upwards for efficacy. Side effects are often a reason for non-compliance and rejection.

Once the drug is chosen, the dosage and frequency can be rapidly increased to achieve:

Maximal relief of symptoms with minimal side effects

Depending on the response, tolerance, and sensitivity of the individual, the drug may have to be changed until the most suitable and effective one is found. Algorithms are only a guide for trial and error. Knowledge of past treatment and familial response is important and also provides useful guidance.

2. **Maintenance Phase**

When the symptoms are relieved or stabilised, side effects may appear unless the dosage and frequency of the drug are reduced. The strategy now is:

Minimal dosage at maximal intervals

3. **Individualisation**

Findings from clinical drug trials are based on "research" diagnosis with standardisation of limited variables and provide only "one size fits all" statistical data, so to speak, for comparison. The usual conclusion is that drug "A" is as efficacious as drug "B". Patients may have the same diagnosis but differ in their response to the same drug and dosage. Therefore, in clinical practice, "tailor-made" management should be the objective. The regime of treatment for each patient is different depending on his symptoms and when they occur, personality variables, family history, daily routine, lifestyle, and other requirements. As most drugs are long acting or have long half-lifes, they are preferably administered in a single dose for instance at night. But if he is doing shift work, he may have to receive his dose when he goes off duty lest he falls asleep at work. Taxi and bus drivers should be closely monitored for side effects. Patients who need to climb when working should be warned of postural hypotension and dizziness; factory operators handling machines should be told of the effects of medication on coordination and reaction time.

Individuals who need to perform well at important functions, such as an interview, taking examinations, and upkeeping public appearance, should find out the **optimal dosage** and **timing** of their medication beforehand. A booster or protective dose may be taken or given in anticipation of stressful changes, environments, life events, and travelling. Any adjustment to medication should preferably be carried out over weekends or holidays to ensure minimal disruption of routines. Taking medicines at work arouses curiosity and invites questions. Therefore, it may be better to prescribe morning and/or evening doses that family members can also help to remind or supervise. When the patient is compliant and stable but relapses, psychosocial factors and changes must be inquired and remedied. Sleep is therapeutic.

Timing of **termination** of treatment depends very much on any significant tasks at hand or events ahead. University studies may be at stake, a career could be in the making, a marriage may be contemplated, a baby could be on the way, someone close may be sick or dying, or an important assignment may have been given. These are potential stressors that can precipitate a relapse, so it is unwise to take unnecessary risks by terminating treatment during such times. On the other hand, a plain-sailing period may never be in view for some patients, so the pros and cons may have to be weighed in order to make a decision.

Past patterns of relapses and remissions should also be considered. In many cases, medication has to be continued indefinitely. When termination is decided, it should be carried out gradually to prevent rebound phenomena or withdrawal symptoms that can be harmful.

Electroconvulsive Therapy

Although **electroconvulsive therapy** (ECT) has been in use since the late 1930s, the treatment is still empirical. It was originally meant for schizophrenia but was subsequently found to be efficacious for **endogenous** or **psychotic depression** and **suicidal** patients. However, ECT has also been prescribed for other conditions because of management problems, such as severely withdrawn and retarded patients who refuse food and drink, excited and aggressive patients who are destructive and in danger of exhausting themselves, and "treatment resistant" patients. ECT is akin to **rebooting** a **computer** that is malfunctioning and unresponsive. The number of sessions of ECT in a course varies from 3–12 or more depending on the severity of conditions and the patient's response. ECT is also sometimes given as "maintenance" for some patients. Meanwhile, medications need to continue.

ECT is a safe procedure when physical fitness is screened and properly carried out. Consent is required from the patient. However, if he/she is unable to give consent, then the LPA/Deputy may give consent or the psychiatrist in charge may, in good faith and in the patient's best interest, order the ECT. Patients are starved, anticonvulsive medications are temporarily omitted, and atropine may sometimes be given to counteract vagal inhibitions on the heart and also reduce secretions during ECT. Short-acting propofol (for general anaesthesia and sedation) and suxamethonium (as a muscle relaxant) are used. In the earlier days, ECT was given "straight" without general anaesthesia, which was frightening and traumatic to the patient. Nowadays, the modified ECT is given with short-acting general anaesthesia and muscle relaxants, and with the anaesthetist in attendance. ECT administration has become rather technical. The principle is to ensure that an optimal current is delivered to induce brain electrical discharge or a seizure (which is therapeutic) has taken place, either from the EEG recording or by observing mild convulsions or twitching for sufficient durations. It is important to realise that paralysis before general anaesthesia sets in is terrifying. Oxygenation or ventilation must be ensured. The threshold of current for the first ECT must also be determined and may be calibrated for subsequent ECTs. The MECTA Spectrum 5000Q ECT machine is used in our neurostimulation services (i.e., ECT and transcranial magnetic stimulation). The choice of bilateral (i.e., bitemporal or bifrontal) or unilateral ECT is recommended according to diagnosis, potential memory disturbance, and handedness. To be therapeutic, the duration of induced seizure should be 25–30 seconds. Too much current will aggravate post-ECT amnesia. ECT is usually administered on alternate days and progress should be reviewed after each ECT to decide on the further course of treatment. It can be given to both inpatients and outpatients.

Side effects like headache, giddiness, and memory impairment are transient or temporary, and complications like fractures and cardiac arrests are rare.

Contraindications include abnormal ECG, recent myocardial infarctions, risk of cerebrovascular accidents, raised intracranial pressure, decompensated pulmonary conditions, and the use of pacemakers.

Transcranial Magnetic Stimulation

Transcranial magnetic stimulation (TMS) is an investigative tool that was first used by neurologists. An electric current is passed through an insulated coil placed on the surface of the scalp. By changing the current through the coil, magnetic fields are generated which stimulate the neurons in the cortex beneath. The magnetic stimulation has the capacity to interrupt and facilitate neuronal functions such as neurotransmission, neurocircuitry, and neuroplasticity probably through depolarisation. In the process of stimulating cortical areas and mapping cortical functions, neurological studies have shown the potential antidepressant effects of TMS. Clinical research is being carried out to establish its therapeutic efficacy for different types of depressive illnesses, OCD, and PTSD. For the latter two, "provocation" to arouse anxiety before giving TMS is necessary.

Deep Brain Stimulation

This involves implanting a "brain pacemaker" that sends electrical impulses through implanted electrodes to specific parts of the brain for relief of treatment-resistant movement, affective disorders, and chronic pains. It is still in the research stage and conditions treated include depression, OCD, Parkinson's disease, essential tremors, Tourette's syndrome, dystonia, and cluster headaches.

Brain Imaging Studies and Research

There has been active and impressive brain imaging studies (e.g., MRI, PET, SPECT) carried out on various psychiatric disorders. Associated functional or dysfunctional areas in the brain have been located. However, there is still a long way to go in interpreting the findings in terms of cause and effect and working out their pathophysiology, psychopathology, and intervention.

Treatment of Schizophrenia

Schizophrenic disorders are characterised by symptoms of hallucination, delusion, thought disorder, abnormal behaviour, blunting of affect, loss of volition, and social withdrawal in varying combinations and proportions. The symptoms may be circumscribed, covert, and intellectualised, or florid, bizarre, and regressive. There is splitting or **disintegration** of mental functions.

In the **dopamine theory** of schizophrenia, it is postulated that schizophrenic symptoms are a result of abnormal levels of dopaminergic activity (hyper or hypo) in the brain. The neuroleptics, which are antipsychotics, act by blocking **postsynaptic dopamine receptors**, particularly D^2, in the **mesolimbic, mesocortical, nigrostriatal**, and **tuberoinfundibular** pathways.

These actions broadly correspond to their **antipsychotic** (mesolimbic), **extra-pyramidal** (nigrostriatal), and **endocrinal or autonomic** effects (e.g., galactorrhoea-amenorrhoea syndrome from increased prolactin levels). In addition, the blocking of dopamine receptors in the **mesocortical** pathway may contribute to or aggravate negative symptoms of schizophrenia and cognitive impairment due to hypo-dopaminergic activity. The clinical picture is similar to the **syndrome of hypo-frontality**.

There are many antipsychotics in the market. Their overall efficacy is about the same and they differ mainly in their side effects profile. The typical or first-generation ones in our practice are chlorpromazine, thioridazine (currently no longer available), trifluoperazine, perphenazine (which are phenothiazines), and haloperidol (which is a butyrophenone). They are also known as major tranquillisers or neuroleptics with strong affinity for the D_2 receptors and hence produce extra-pyramidal symptoms (EPS). Second-generation **atypical antipsychotics** are characterised by their weaker or moderate affinity for D_2 receptors and are also antagonists of **$5HT_2$** receptors. They have less or minimal EPS and also ameliorate negative symptoms. This could be due to the release of dopamine through disinhibition when $5HT_2$ receptors are blocked. Another postulation is that there is "**rapid dissociation**" from or "**transient occupation**" of the dopamine receptors (i.e., clozapine and quetiapine). The **$5HT_2$** receptors may also have a role in psychosis. These atypical antipsychotics are believed to act differentially on the dopaminergic system (i.e., in the prefrontal cortex) to improve cognitive functioning (with antidepressant effect), in the basal ganglia to reduce EPS, and in the tuberoinfundibular system to check on prolactin secretion. This class of newer antipsychotics includes **clozapine**, **risperidone**, **olanzapine**, **quetiapine**, and **ziprasidone**. **Amisulpride** has no affinity for $5HT_2$ receptors but is alleged to be atypical too because it improves negative symptoms and has less EPS. Although the benefits of atypical antipsychotics are reduced EPS and improvement of negative symptoms, they have been found in recent years to be associated with the development of metabolic disturbances leading to **weight gain**, **diabetes mellitus**, and **hyperlipidaemia** (especially clozapine and olanzapine), perhaps in those predisposed, to various degrees. Due to blocked serotonin receptors, obsessive-compulsive symptoms may result (e.g., risperidone and clozapine).

Chlorpromazine and **thioridazine** are more sedative (i.e., causing drowsiness) and better indicated for excited and disturbed patients. They are prescribed in multiples of 25 mg. The dosage is from 25 mg to 100 mg three times per day or more (e.g., 1g daily in divided doses). Common side effects include drowsiness, postural hypotension, weakness, and constipation. Thioridazine is strongly anticholinergic and may be toxic to the heart (i.e., causing arrhythmia). In addition, nasal congestion is often complained of. Although safe when used judiciously, its supply has been **stopped** by the manufacturer. In mega doses of antipsychotics, ECG may show a **prolonged Q-T interval** and ought to be monitored.

Trifluoperazine and **haloperidol** do not cause much drowsiness but may be more likely to produce extra-pyramidal disturbances. Trifluoperazine seems better indicated for more withdrawn patients and those with hallucinatory and delusional symptoms. It is given from 5 mg two twice per day to 10 mg thrice per day. Haloperidol is better indicated for more manic patients and is given from 1.5 mg twice per day to 5–10 mg thrice per day. It has a long half-life and side effects like stiffness, pains, and aches, and akathisia may last for weeks even after discontinuation.

When the acute stage is over, the daily drug dosage can be reduced to a smaller dose in the morning and a larger dose in the evening, or just one big single dose at night. It must be mentioned that typical antipsychotics can induce weight gain and obesity.

Antipsychotics in colourless, odourless, and tasteless **liquid** form are available. This is very useful for patients who have difficulty swallowing tablets or need careful titration. It is also used in patients who are uncooperative, resistive, and suspicious. The drops can be added into drinks, soup, or food. However, caution should be exercised in prescription and usage in case of abuse and breach of **ethics**. Liquid haloperidol, clopixol, and risperidone are available. Covert treatment is now disallowed due to ethics and rights.

Other drugs like **pimozide, sulpiride**, and **amisulpride** are said to have less extra-pyramidal side effects. Pimozide 1–4 mg every night was once recommended for monosymptomatic hypochondriacal psychosis. It is long acting and can cause cardiac arrhythmias. **Sulpiride** has been used more for anxiety and hypochondriacal symptoms than as an antipsychotic. However, in **liaison** psychiatry, it is considered as carrying lower or moderate risk in pregnancy, breast feeding, cardiovascular disease, diabetes, epilepsy, liver disease, and renal impairment. The dosage ranges from 100 to 600 mg a day. **Amisulpride** acts on D_2 and D_3 receptors. In low doses such as 50–100 mg/day, it stimulates the pre-synaptic autoreceptors to release dopamine, which ameliorates negative symptoms probably through the mesocortical pathway. At higher doses such as 600–800 mg/day, it blocks the postsynaptic receptors in the mesolimbic pathway to suppress positive symptoms. The medium range of 400–600 mg/day controls both positive and negative symptoms of schizophrenia.

In old and frail patients, risperidone 0.25–0.5 mg, amisulpride 50 mg, olanzapine 2.5 mg, or quetiapine 12.5–25 mg can be prescribed. However, side effects like anticholinergic and extrapyramidal symptoms must be avoided or minimised.

Clozapine, discovered in 1959 and launched in the early 1970s, was withdrawn a few years later because of fatal **agranulocytosis** (without granulocytes; i.e., neutrophils, eosinophils, basophils) or **granulopenia** (marked decrease in granulocytes). But in the late 1980s, it was revived and repackaged to treat so-called **treatment resistant** (or treatment refractory) schizophrenics and/or those who are greatly troubled by extra-pyramidal symptoms. Negative symptoms are also improved. The term "treatment resistant" is misleading unless qualified by "to what"? If clozapine is prescribed as a first-line antipsychotic for schizophrenia, then only two thirds or so treated would respond and the rest would be treatment resistant to clozapine. Clozapine has its own side effects such as sedation, salivation (M4), seizures, cardiac toxicity, anticholinergic and antihistaminergic effects, hypotension, central nervous system and metabolic disturbances, and most importantly (non-dose-related) **agranulocytosis**, which occurs in about **<1%** of patients mostly during the first 6 months. Regular monitoring of white blood cells (WBC) and absolute neutrophils count (ANC), weekly for the first 18 weeks and later fortnightly for 6 months and thereafter monthly, must be carried out to avoid potential fatality. To be safe, the patient should have a **WBC of >3500 mm^3** and **ANC of >2000 mm^3** and be free from infection and fever (lithium and ascorbic acid are thought to protect leucopenia). Clozapine has minimal or no extra-pyramidal symptoms and the improvement rate of the so-called "treatment resistant" cases are between one and two thirds.

More recently, clozapine has also been reported to be promising in the treatment of suicidality in schizophrenia, aggression in psychotic patients, schizophrenia with polydipsia and hyponatraemia, refractory and psychotic depression, and mania. It is also sometimes used in the treatment of tardive dyskinesia. However, the use of clozapine should best be left to **specialists**. The dosage should be titrated gradually upwards from 25 mg daily.

Risperidone is effective against both **positive** and **negative** schizophrenic symptoms and dose dependent extra-pyramidal side effects (**EPSE**) may develop at the higher end. The dosage should be titrated gradually and slowly from 0.5–1 mg a day up to 4–6 mg daily. Due to serotonin blockade, **serotonin-related syndromes** (e.g., obsessive-compulsive symptoms, apathetic depression, weight gain, sexual dysfunction) may develop. Adjustment of dosage and adjunct medications may be necessary. Incidence of stroke in elderly patients has also been reported.

Paliperidone is a recently registered antipsychotic. It is actually the main active metabolite of risperidone, undergoes minimal hepatic biotransformation, and is excreted mainly unchanged in the urine. As such, it is similar in efficacy and side effects as risperidone. However, it comes as a once-a-day, extended release preparation capsule of 3 mg, 6 mg, 9 mg, or 12 mg. The osmotic controlled-release oral delivery system provides a steady therapeutic level, thus minimising peak-trough fluctuation. A dosage of 6 mg should be sufficient.

Olanzapine resembles clozapine in chemical structure and pharmacological profile. Its plasma half-life is about 30 hours and a single dose of 5–10 mg/day is prescribed. Although efficacious for positive and negative symptoms of schizophrenia, it carries a higher risk of weight gain, increase in plasma glucose level, type II diabetes, and lipidaemia. Its sedative action may be better indicated for more agitated and manic patients.

Quetiapine interacts with broad range of neurotransmitter receptors. It has a short half-life of 3–6 hours and no active metabolites. Therefore, it is prescribed as 150–600 mg/day to be taken twice or thrice a day. In practice however, a single dose daily seems effective. It is low in extra-pyramidal symptoms, tardive dyskinesia, weight gain, and hyperglycaemia when compared with clozapine and olanzapine. It is useful for elderly patients with psychotic disorders and drug-induced psychosis in Parkinson's disease, and 25 mg a day may be sufficient. In low doses, it may have antidepressant and anti-anxiety properties.

Other marketed atypical antipsychotics include sertindole and ziprasidone. **Sertindole** has the longest elimination half-life of about 3 days among the atypical antipsychotics. It seems to act mainly on the limbic system. The dosage is 4–12 mg daily or more. Its effect on QTc prolongation is similar to thioridazine and pimoside. **Ziprasidone** comes in both oral (given 40 mg twice a day) and injection form. The latter seems to be more sedative. It is claimed to cause less weight gain, hyperglycaemia, and hyper-cholesterol. Together with quetiapine and clozapine, it causes less prolactin elevation.

Neurotransmitter receptor affinities and effects

	D_2 (antipsychotic)	$5HT_{2A}$ (D release)	$Alpha_1$ (orthostatic)	M_1 (anticholinergic)	H_1 (antihistamine)
Clozapine	++(L)	++++	++++	++++	++++
Risperidone	++++	++++	++++	--	++
Olanzapine	++(L)	++++	++	++++	++++
Quetiapine	++	++	++	++	++++
Ziprasidone	++	++++	++	--	+/-
Sertindole	+++(L)	+++	++	--	+

Depending on the source of reference, varying data are quoted by different authors. Drugs with H_1 affinity contribute to sedation and weight gain. However, there may be other reasons besides H_1 affinity for weight gain, such as $5HT_{2C}$ pathway, satiety centre dysfunction, slow metabolism, and insulin resistance, induced or otherwise. Susceptible individuals include young patients, women, psychotic mood disorder patients, and those with family history of similar responses.

Rapid switching or sudden withdrawal of drugs may precipitate rebound symptoms according to the neurotransmitters and receptor affinities involved. Therefore, when switching from one drug to another, dovetailing is advisable (i.e., gradual decrease of one and increase of the other).

Aripiprazole, a dopamine partial agonist, is a recently available atypical antipsychotic. It functions as a **partial agonist** when there is hypo-dopaminergic activity (i.e., in the **mesocortical** pathway) and functions as a postsynaptic **antagonist** at D_2 receptors when there is hyper-dopaminergic activity (i.e. in the **mesolimbic** pathway). In addition, it is also a partial agonist to $5HT_{1A}$ and an antagonist of $5HT_{2A}$ receptors, which increases DA release in the prefrontal cortex and NE transmission respectively. It has been described as a third-generation antipsychotic that is efficacious for both positive and negative symptoms. However, a Cochrane review found weak evidence of efficacy for treatment of schizophrenia. It is also claimed to have a better side effects profile (i.e., less sedation, but may cause insomnia and headache), less extra-pyramidal symptoms, anticholinergic side effects, hypotension, and hyperprolactinaemia, and also less risk of weight gain, adverse changes in glucose metabolism, lipids, and ECGs when compared with other atypical antipsychotics. It is prescribed in 10 or 15 mg every morning, although the dosage should be halved when fluoxetine or paroxetine is concomitantly prescribed. It has also been used empirically as an adjunct for treatment resistant OCD as well as major depressive disorder. However, compulsive behaviour (e.g., gambling) has been noted. **Brexpiprazole** like aripiprazole is a serotonin and dopamine activity modulator for the treatment of schizophrenia and depression, but with lesser affinity for D_2 and D_3 and greater affinity for $5HT_{1A}$, $5HT_{2A}$, and alpha 1B with consequent actions and effects. The optimal dosage for schizophrenia is 1–4 mg a day and <2 mg daily for MDD.

In some patients treated with atypical antipsychotics, although their symptoms of delusion and hallucination may persist, they somehow seem more tolerant of them and do not respond or react as strongly as before.

Based on the hypothesis of hypo-frontality (due perhaps to reduced dopaminergic activity in the mesocortical pathway), **amineptine** (a dopaminergic antidepressant) 50–100 mg is given every morning to those with negative symptoms, though some positive symptoms were reactivated. However, due to the potential for dependency, the drug has been withdrawn. Conversely, for schizophrenic patients who are florid in symptoms, impulsive, suicidal, and violent, addition of **escitalopram** 5–10 mg taken at night seems to help. It appears to dampen behavioural responses to psychotic symptoms, such as delusion and hallucination. However, it may also trigger hypomanic symptoms.

Asenapine is one of the latest **atypical antipsychotics** with high affinity for serotonin, adrenaline, dopamine, and histamine and low affinity for muscarinic acetylcholine receptors. It is a partial agonist at $5HT_{1A}$ receptors and an antagonist to others. It is indicated for schizophrenia and bipolar mania and claims to have less anti-cholinergic and cardiovascular side effects and weight gains. However, like the other antipsychotics, it may have side effects like akathisia, oral hypoaesthesia somnolence, extra-pyramidal symptoms, or metabolic disturbance. It is not recommended for psychotic symptoms in dementia. The tablet should be taken dry, whole, and sublingually followed by no food and drink for 10 minutes. The dosage is 5–10 mg twice per day. Drug interactions and effects on liver functions should be noted.

Depot Injections

Long-acting antipsychotic drugs are not only useful in patients who are non-compliant with medication but also to those who may not respond well to oral medications with reduced bio-availability in the gut and liver. There are many depot injections available. In general, one dose is given 2–4 times weekly or longer depending on the state of remission and stability of illness and is often fine-tuned with oral medications. Dosage varies with the severity of illness, efficacy, and side effects. Duration and timing are flexible rather than fixed and according to anticipation of life events, presence of high expressed emotions, and intensity of physical and psychosocial activities and factors. It is not unlike charging a smartphone according to usage, reserves available, and anticipated use. There are many long-acting depot antipsychotics available now in IMH/WH.

Fluphenazine decanoate (Modecate)

Fluphenazine decanoate is the earliest typical antipsychotic depot injection. It is generic, effective, cheap, and comes in both vial and ampoule forms. The disadvantages commonly complained of are extra-pyramidal side effects and depression. However, when properly prescribed and monitored, they can be minimised. Regrettably, its production and promotion has been limited.

To illustrate the principles of prescription, 12.5 mg may be given weekly during the acute stage when the patient is in the hospital. Usually, 6.25 mg (1/4 ml) is started off as the "test" dose. The maintenance dose is quite variable, ranging from 6.25 mg 6–8 times weekly to 50 mg twice weekly. Experienced patients are able to judge for themselves when the effect of the drug is wearing off and will often come before the appointment date for an earlier injection. The dosage and the interval should be flexible and adjusted according to the needs and convenience of the patient. When there is more mental activity, social interaction, or stressful events, more of the drug will be needed. It is not unlike a battery that needs to be frequently recharged when overused. On the other hand, when life is quiet and peaceful, less medication is required. The same principles apply to the other depots.

Pipothiazine palmitate (Piportil)

This comes in 50 mg ampoules and is administered 12.5–50 mg each time. It is thought to have less side effects and is possibly effective for a longer interval. However, it is costly and regrettably not available now.

Flupentixol decanoate (Fluanxol)

This comes in 20 mg and 40 mg ampoules. Besides being an antipsychotic, it has also been claimed to have antidepressant properties at lower dosages. A recent finding is that it has affinity for D_2 as well as $5HT_2$ receptors. As such, it is like the "atypical" antipsychotics that are efficacious for schizophrenia with positive and negative symptoms and have less side effects. It has been recommended by some reports for patients who are repeatedly suicidal probably because of some antidepressant effect.

Zuclopenthixol decanoate (Clopixol)

This typical antipsychotic comes in 200 mg ampoules and is recommended for patients who tend to be aggressive or violent. 200–400 mg can be given once every 2–4 weeks. Liquid form is available and given in drops like haloperidol liquid. Recent personal experience suggests that it ameliorates regressive thinking and speech or behaviours that are illogical, irrational, irrelevant, or "nonsensical".

Risperidone (Consta)

Risperidone differs from the other depots in that the first dose takes about 3 weeks to be effective. The patient therefore needs to continue with the oral risperidone or antipsychotic during this period. The starting dose is 25 mg and can be increased to 37.5 mg or 50 mg later. The depot side effects are reportedly less than the oral risperidone. It is recommended to be given 2 to probably 4 times weekly. The cost of consta 25 mg and 37.5 mg per ampoule are several times that of typical antipsychotic depots.

Haloperidol decanoate

The depot comes in 100 mg/ml ampoule. It is non-standard and yet to be fully registered by the HSA. Like "consta", oral antipsychotics (e.g., haloperidol) must be continued for 2 to 4 weeks when initiating the depot because the absorption rate constant is slower than the elimination rate constant. The depot has a slightly longer half-life than the oral haloperidol. The conversion dosage is roughly 100 mg four times per week depot, which is equivalent to chlorpromazine

500 mg daily. The initial dose of 50 mg depot is about 10–15 times the daily dose of oral haloperidol. The maintenance dose is 50–200 mg 2–6 times weekly (see principles under "modecate").

Paliperidone palmitate

This is a new atypical antipsychotic depot. It is supposed to be non-sedative, non-anticholinergic, and low in extra-pyramidal symptoms and metabolic disturbance. It is used in non-acute patients with schizophrenia and claims of superior remission. The trade name Invega Sustena comes in 50 mg, 75 mg, 100 mg, and 150 mg PR INJ (monthly) and the Invega Trinza comes in 175 mg, 263 mg, 350 mg, and 525 mg PR INJ (3 monthly). They cost a few hundred to over a thousand dollars per dose. For the Invega Sustena, the initial regiment is 150 mg on Day 1 injected into the deltoid, 100mg on Day 8 injected into the deltoid, 75 mg on Day 38 (+/– 7 days) injected into the deltoid or gluteal, and thereafter 4 times weekly (+/– 7 days) injected into the deltoid or gluteal based on pharmacokinetics. After three consecutive months of Invega Sustena, the thrice monthly Invega Trinza can be given with an equivalent dosage recommended. Paliperidone is a metabolite of risperidone and is excreted by the kidneys. In the initial stage, an anti-anxiety or sedative drug may be needed. While switching over from more sedative antipsychotics, tailing off should be gradual.

Aripiprazol 400 mg INJ (Abilify Maintena)

Aripiprazol is a recent addition to the list of antipsychotic depot injections (see aripiprazole).

Adjunct Medication

As symptoms of anxiety and depression are present in many psychotic disorders, they can be treated with SSRIs to reduce exacerbation and aggravation of mental symptoms. Anecdotally, in some schizophrenic patients, SSRIs seem to reduce psychotic hallucinations and delusions, which may be expressions of **subconscious** or **unconscious** obsessional ruminations **not recognised** by the conscious mind. Or perhaps due to drug interactions, the SSRI might have enhanced the effect of the antipsychotic used. They are also added to relieve obsessive-compulsive symptoms (e.g., suicidal rumination, trichotillomania, compulsive ritual induced by atypical antipsychotic drugs) because of their $5HT_2$ blocking action. Tianeptine appears useful in protecting against relapse from high expressed emotion and stress.

Side Effects of Neuroleptics

One should be familiar with the many possible side effects of neuroleptics or antipsychotics. Distressing side effects are a major reason for non-compliance with medications. Apart from the more dramatic oculogyric crisis, dystonia, and Parkinsonism, there are frequent complaints of giddiness or dizziness, drowsiness, weakness, headaches, muscular pains, tremors, dryness of mouth, blurring of vision, constipation, nausea, increased appetite, weight gain, amenorrhoea, and sexual dysfunction. There may also be allergic reactions, seizures, and blood dyscrasia. However, the same drug may not always induce the same side effects or allergic reactions in the same patient. When necessary, the drug can be used again and titrated all over.

Two other side effects are particularly important. **Tardive dyskinesia** (TD), or the involuntary movements of the tongue, mouth, jaw, trunk, and/or limbs (after prolonged medication) are socially embarrassing if not personally distressing. Repeated belching may be due to diaphragmatic TD. As there is no specific remedy, it is something that is best prevented by reducing the use of neuroleptics and avoiding or withdrawing anti-Parkinsonism drugs whenever possible. The other serious side effect is **akathisia**, which is a most distressing symptom that can drive a patient to suicide or violent behaviour. The patient complains of extreme uneasiness and restlessness. They are unable to keep still for long and move about. A milder and transient complaint may occur towards evening. Not infrequently, neuroleptics are mistakenly stepped up rather than reduced or stopped. Propranolol, diazepam, and mirtazapine may help to ameliorate the symptom.

In acute **dystonia** with spasm and pain, symptoms can be relieved with diazepam 10 mg, benzhexol (artane) 2 mg, and adjustment of the neuroleptics. In the case of oculogyric crisis, i/m diphenhydramine 25–50 mg or i/m benztropine (cogentin) 1–2 mg can be given followed by oral benzhexol and a review of medication. As it tends to recur usually towards the evening, it is better to prescribe benzhexol 2 mg prophylactically at about 4 p.m. rather than at night, apart from the morning dose. **Spasmodic torticollis** can be relieved by oral diphenhydramine.

Neuroleptic Malignant Syndrome (NMS)

Neuroleptic malignant syndrome (NMS) is a **serious** and **potentially fatal complication** from neuroleptic medication. Patients usually develop NMS during the first two weeks after antipsychotic treatment. **Clinical features** include muscle rigidity, clouding of consciousness, hyperpyrexia, leukocytosis, tachycardia, labile blood pressure, and elevated creatinine phosphokinase (similar to the combined features of catatonia, infection, and autonomic dysfunction). The patient may go into a coma and die of cardio-respiratory and renal failures. Possible risk factors include male gender, organic brain disease, mental retardation, rapid neuroleptisation, and concomitant lithium therapy.

In management, **early detection** of restlessness, mild rigidity, and low-grade fever with prompt discontinuation of antipsychotic medication may avert a full-blown syndrome. Intensive supportive medical care, the muscle relaxant **dantrolene**, and the dopamine agonist **bromocriptine** have been found to be efficacious. Benzodiazepines may also be helpful in reversing the condition.

Anti-Parkinsonism Drug

Benzhexol Hydrochloride (Artane)

This anti-Parkinsonism preparation is highly addictive and in demand by abusers. It is also believed to predispose and aggravate tardive dyskinesia. When taken in excess, the patient may develop toxic symptoms, such as flushing with hyperpyrexia, tachycardia, dilation of pupils with blurring of vision, and even delirium. It should therefore be prescribed sparingly and only when indicated. However, one should balance complete omission with the risk of default on treatment because of unpleasant extra-pyramidal side effects from neuroleptic medications. In outpatient settings, it may be better to give a small dose of artane for a short period of time. When no unpleasant extra-pyramidal side effects are reported, then it should be withdrawn quickly. For patients on depot neuroleptics, artane may be prescribed for the first one to two weeks when the side effects are most likely to appear. For urgent relief of acute extra-pyramidal side effects, injection of cogentin 2 mg or diphenhydramine 25–50 mg is available. Oral **benztropine** may be used in place of benzhexol.

Treatment of Affective Disorders

Antidepressants

Antidepressants may be grouped under monoamine reuptake inhibitors (TCAs; e.g., tricyclic antidepressants), monoamines oxidase inhibitors (MAOIs; e.g., phenelzine and moclobemide which is a reversible MAOI), selective serotonin reuptake inhibitors (SSRIs), and the more recently promoted serotonin and noradrenaline reuptake inhibitors (SNRIs, NaSSA). They are also efficacious for anxiety disorders.

In depression, the hypothesis is that there is a deficiency of noradrenaline, dopamine, and serotonin neurotransmitters in the synaptic junctions. The action of MAOIs is to increase the synthesis and storage of noradrenaline and dopamine in the presynaptic neurons. The reuptake inhibitors act essentially on presynaptic transporters (reuptake pumps) to increase the availability of monoamines for neurotransmission. The different reuptake inhibitors also act on different postsynaptic receptors to produce or block different side effects and perhaps enhance therapeutic efficacy. The amount of noradrenaline, dopamine, or serotonin in the synaptic junction is also regulated by the feedback mechanisms of the respective presynaptic autoreceptors that control its release. These monoamines then act on appropriate postsynaptic receptors to achieve therapeutic results, but also on some other receptors to cause side effects.

The **TCAs** are noradrenaline, serotonin, and dopamine agonists in varying degrees and most of them have rather troublesome **anticholinergic** side effects that can be quite intolerable. Otherwise, they are potent antidepressants. The common TCAs include amitriptyline, imipramine, trimipramine, clomipramine, and dothiepin. They are prescribed in multiples of 25 mg, ranging from 25 mg to 150 mg in divided doses, or one single dose at night as they are also sedative and can double up as hypnotics as well.

Amitriptyline is comparatively more sedative and, given its cardiotoxicity, can be fatal in an overdose. **Clomipramine**, which is the most serotonergic among the TCAs, is commonly used for obsessive-compulsive disorder. **Imipramine** is also frequently prescribed for phobic anxiety syndrome (e.g., agoraphobia and panic disorder). **Dothiepin** appears to be fast acting and improvement can be seen early. **ECG** monitoring for prolonged Q-T interval is advisable.

It is good practice to inform patients of possible side effects during the initial period of treatment and that it takes two to three weeks before they begin to feel better. Common **side effects** of standard **TCAs** include giddiness, drowsiness, dryness of mouth, constipation, acute retention of urine, impotence, blurring of vision, and sweating. They are often the reasons for default on treatment. Therefore, dosage ought to be built up gradually and reviewed at short intervals until optimal results are achieved. **Contraindications** include glaucoma, enlarged prostate, and ischaemic heart disease.

Mianserin, maprotiline, and **nortriptyline** are heterocyclic antidepressants. Mianserin may cause drowsiness; maprotiline may lower seizure threshold; and nortriptyline is contraindicated in patients with heart conditions. They are not often in use nowadays. **Flupentixol** in small doses is claimed to have antidepressant properties.

For patients with known cardiac conditions (abnormal ECGs) and those who are unable to tolerate anticholinergic side effects, the newer SSRIs are preferred. Mianserin and moclobemide can also be prescribed.

The newer **SSRIs** are said to have mild or little anticholinergic side effects and less cardiotoxicity. There are four main **serotonin pathways** in the central nervous system (cf., dopaminergic pathways) through which serotonin is released simultaneously when serotonin neurons are disinhibited. The pathways are from the midbrain raphe to (i) the **prefrontal cortex**, (ii) **basal ganglia**, (iii) **limbic cortex** and **hippocampus**, and (iv) **hypothalamus**. The desired **5HT$_{1A}$** actions (on both presynaptic and postsynaptic receptors) of SSRIs may be said to correspond to their therapeutic effects on **depression, obsessive-compulsive disorder, panic disorder**, and **bulimia** respectively. On the other hand, they may also cause side effects such as anxiety, agitation, akathisia, panic attacks, insomnia, and sexual dysfunction due to stimulation of **5HT$_2$** receptors as well as nausea, GI distress, diarrhoea, and headache due to stimulation of **5HT$_3$** receptors (these side effects probably constitute the "serotonin syndrome" described).

Thus, **fluoxetine** may cause nervousness, anxiety, insomnia, and impotence and is better indicated for the more retarded. It should be taken in doses of 10–40 mg in the morning with or without an adjunct benzodiazepine. The dispersible tablet form is recently available and it has a long half-life of 2–3 days, the longest among the SSRIs. It is preferably indicated for young patients. **Fluvoxamine** is given in doses of 50–100 mg twice a day or up to 100–200 mg at night as it could be sedative. Some consider it the drug of choice for obsessive-compulsive disorder, but some patients complain of gastric discomfort. **Paroxetine** should be started with 10–20 mg every morning and gradually increased by 10 mg to 40 mg daily. It seems to work well for the more "**neurotic**" depression and anxiety disorders. Withdrawal should be gradual. **Sertraline** has a similar dosage range as fluvoxamine, but the optimal dosage recommended is 50 mg daily due to gastric symptoms. It is also dopaminergic and better indicated for concomitant Parkinsonism. **Escitalopram** can be given 5–10 mg at night or 2.5–5 mg twice per day as it can be sedative as well as effective in improving poor control of impulses that may be aggressive or suicidal. It is fast acting and also a relatively safe drug to use when there are concomitant medical conditions, such as cardiac, liver, or renal problems.

Mirtazapine (NaSSA), an alpha-2 antagonist, is a noradrenergic and specific serotonergic antidepressant. It not only increases the release of noradrenaline and serotonin and enhances their neurotransmission via $5HT_{1A}$ but also blocks $5HT_2$ and $5HT_3$ and their unwanted side effects. However, due to its antihistamine properties, there may be drowsiness and weight gain. It is useful in promoting sleep and appetite. The dosage is 15–30 mg every night but the sedation may be inversely related to dosage. It may augment conventional antipsychotics to simulate an atypical antipsychotic or ameliorate its induced akathisia. **Venlafaxine** at low doses inhibits reuptake of serotonin and in increasingly higher doses inhibits noradrenaline and then dopamine. Due to its short half-life, it is given from 25 mg to 50 mg twice per day. A slow release 75 mg tablet/day is available. Elderly patients may experience hypertension. **Trazadone** is a serotonin antagonist and a partial agonist of $5HT_{1A}$ and has both antidepressant and anxiolytic effects but little anticholinergic side effects. It is sedative and therefore better indicated for depression with anxiety, agitation, and insomnia. The somnolent effect probably results from excessive $5HT_2$ blockade. The dosage ranges from 100–300 mg daily in divided doses. **Duloxetine** is a recent dual action (i.e., noradrenaline and serotonin) agonist antidepressant. Its efficacy and side effects are comparable to other antidepressants. However, its purported ability to relieve somatised pain and neuropathic pain in diabetes mellitus has not been studied in the other antidepressants. It is given as a single 30–60 mg dose daily. It is contraindicated in patients with liver conditions.

As a rule, **MAOIs** should not be used together with other anti-depressants because the release of synthesised monoamines from presynaptic terminals will increase the concentration of mono-amines in the synaptic junctions, causing untoward reactions such as acute rise of blood pressure which may be fatal. Therefore, when switching over from MAOIs to TCAs, a **washout** period of two weeks is required.

Tianeptine (**Stablon**) is a novel antidepressant with anti-anxiety effects. Unlike SSRIs, it enhances the reuptake of sero-tonin, dampens the **hypothalamopituitary adrenocortical** (HPA) axis stress response, and protects or restores hippocampal CA1 and CA3 pyramidal cells from stress-induced toxic effects and dysfunction, albeit in rats. It is debatable whether the antidepres-sant efficacy is via the reuptake of serotonin. Its therapeutic effi-cacy is probably best indicated for **stress-induced** symptoms or disorders of which insomnia, anxiety, and depression are the most common. It also **protects** patients with schizophrenia (or perhaps recurrent affective disorder), who are exposed to high expressed emotions of stressful or high arousal environments, from relaps-ing. The side effects are mild, including gastric discomfort, sleepi-ness, and possibly obsessional rumination. The dosage varies from 12.5mg two or three times daily.

Patients may try **bupropion**, a noradrenaline and dopamine reuptake inhibitor, and **buspirone**, a $5HT_{1A}$ partial agonist, for SSRI-induced sexual dysfunction and as an adjunct antidepressant for refractory depression. Bupropion is also prescribed for smok-ing cessation, but it may induce auditory hallucinations and cause insomnia. Buspirone has been used to treat anxiety disorders.

In the treatment of depression, both the **symptoms profile** of the patient and the **pharmacological profile** of the drug must be taken into consideration. Different antidepressants may have to be trialed for efficacy and side effects. Treatment should normally continue for some months after recovery or relief of symptoms as relapse is common if medication is stopped too soon. The recent trend is to maintain the medication at a therapeutic level rather than at a lower maintenance level. It is sometimes even advocated that treatment should be prolonged for an indefinite period of time. This may be necessary and correct, but it is unclear whether this is due to the **nature of the illness** (endogenous or exogenous) or that some **perpetuating psychosocial stressors** have been ignored. The latter seems more likely as it should be common sense that the patient is not going to recover insofar as the psychosocial stressors persist. Medication is no substitute for appropriate intervention and resolution of psychosocial stressors when indicated. One in six depressed (bipolar) patients may commit suicide (see also the relations between anxiety and depression).

Like schizophrenia, there are depressed patients who do not respond to the usual antidepressants. Such patients are managed by specialists with various combinations of antidepressants or augmented with lithium and anticonvulsants (i.e., carbamazepine, sodium valproate, and lamotrigine), in particular unipolar or bipolar depression. When combining SSRIs and TCAs in the treatment of **refractory depression**, it is important to bear in mind drug interactions. The liver **cytochrome P450** (CYP) superfamily of enzymes is involved in most drug metabolism. SSRIs (in particular fluoxetine, paroxetine and less so sertraline and escitalopram) **inhibit CYP 2D6** which metabolises TCAs, antipsychotics, antiarrythmics, and beta blockers, thus increasing their plasma levels and causing toxic effects. Fluvoxamine inhibits both **CYP 1A2** and **CYP 3A4**, which eliminate warfarin, TCAs, clozapine, benzodiazepines, and some antiarrythmics. Drug dosages should therefore be adjusted or reduced. Escitalopram is relatively free from hepatic interaction. Empirically, **lamotrigine** seems promising in the treatment of protracted or bipolar depression. It has to be given very gradually and starting from a very low dose. Rashes or skin eruptions may occur and cleft palate incidence has recently been reported when given during pregnancy.

Treatment with antidepressants can lead to SIADH and **hyponatraemia** with complaints of dizziness, nausea, lethargy, confusion, cramps, and seizures. Baseline and follow up serum sodium should be determined. **Lately**, there has been **caution on suicide risk** when prescribing new generation antidepressants such as SSRIs for children and adolescents in particular. While rates of actual suicide have yet to be documented, there appears to be an **increased occurrence** of suicidal ideation and behaviour. This "alarming warning" is probably based on anecdotal reports and questionnaire surveys, but no explanation is given for the finding. Could it be that depression has been so **over-diagnosed** and **over-treated** that patients suffer from distressing and intolerable side effects? Could the lack of efficacy of the antidepressants (in one third or more) be causing the depression to truly express itself? Could predisposing and propagating environmental factors have been overlooked and ignored? Whatever the implications, there should be a balance between potential medico-legal liability and realistic clinical practice.

Agomelatine

This is a relatively new antidepressant that is an agonist to the melatonin receptors MT_1/MT_2 and an antagonist to the serotonin receptor $5HT_{2C}$. It claims to be efficacious in treating major depression by **resynchronising** the disturbed **circadian rhythm**, which is both the cause and result of depressive illness. It restores normal sleep and is efficacious on anhedonia. The side effects are said to be no different from that of placebo. Baseline liver function tests show that the effects on liver enzymes are not significant. The dosage recommended is 25–50 mg daily.

Vortioxetine (Brintellix)

Vortioxetine is a new multimodal antidepressant with a novel mechanism of action that combines direct activity at multiple serotonin receptors. It has agonistic properties at $5HT_{1A}$ with potent inhibition of the serotonin reuptake transporter, and has been approved by the FDA for the treatment of major depressive disorder. Depending on depression rating scales used, it has been claimed to be particularly efficacious for the recovery of cognitive function in depression. The dosage recommended is from 5 mg to 20 mg daily. The side effects consist mainly of gut symptoms like nausea, vomiting, diarrhea, constipation, and dizziness. Sexual side effects were said to be low and similar to placebo. Serotonin syndrome apparently has been reported. Due to its long half-life, rebound phenomenon is unlikely.

Serotonin Syndrome

Serotonin syndrome, like neuroleptic malignant syndrome, is a potentially life-threatening adverse drug reaction that results from the therapeutic use of SSRIs (or proserotonergic agents like nefazodone), intentional self-poisoning, or inadvertent interactions between drugs (e.g., meperidine and phenelzine). In fact, a large number of drugs and drug combinations, including all classes of antidepressants, opiate analgesics, cough mixtures (e.g., dextromethorphan), antimigraine agents (e.g., sumatriptan), drugs of abuse (e.g., LSD, ecstasy), anticonvulsants (e.g., valproate), and others (e.g., trytophan, ginseng, lithium) have been associated with the syndrome.

The occurrence of serotonin syndrome requires one to be **aware** of the predictable consequences of excess serotonergic agonists of the central nervous system and peripheral serotonergic receptors. This excess serotonin produces a spectrum of clinical findings and the clinical manifestations of serotonin syndrome range from barely perceptible to lethal. The **onset** is **rapid** in terms of **hours** (cf., **NMS** in **days**) and the **clinical triad** often described consists of:

a. mental state changes — e.g., anxiety, agitation, akathisia, hypervigilance, delirium, coma
b. autonomic hyperactivity — e.g., tremors, shivering, diarrhoea, increased bowel sounds, tachycardia/tachypnoea, excessive sweating (diaphoresis), dilatation of pupils (mydriasis), hypertension
c. neuromuscular abnormalities — e.g., rigidity, hyper-reflexia, clonus/myoclonus (more in lower extremities), hyperthermia, seizure

Management of serotonin syndrome

Precipitating agents should be stopped, although withdrawal of medications such as risperidone (a strong $5HT_2$ antagonist) may be associated with the syndrome. This alone may suffice in mild cases, but because the $5HT_{2A}$ receptors are believed to be involved in more severe cases, cyproheptadine (a $5HT_{2A}$ antagonist) is empirically recommended. A starting oral dose of 10–12 mg is given and subsequently 2 mg 2 hourly pro re nata (i.e., at the patient's discretion). The maintenance is 8 mg 6 hourly.

Symptomatic and supportive treatments for anxiety, clonus/ myoclonus, hyperthermia, tachycardia, and hypertension with benzodiazepines and others are essential.

Antimanics (see WFSBP's recommendation for bipolar disorders)

In local practice for initial manic episodes during the acute disturbed stage, **haloperidol** has been the first-line drug that is often used. Liquid or intra-muscular haloperidol 5–10 mg may be given at intervals in the absence of extra-pyramidal symptoms to achieve stabilisation of behaviour. When the patient is cooperative, oral medication should be started from 1.5 mg to 5 mg thrice per day or up to 10 mg thrice per day. **Lorazepam** 0.5–1 mg thrice per day is recommended. **Chlorpromazine** may be prescribed in addition or on its own from 100–200 mg thrice per day or more. **Clonazepam** 0.5 mg thrice per day has been used as adjunct, but alternatively **diazepam** 5–10 mg or more thrice per day can be given. More recently, there has been an increasing promotion of the atypical antipsychotics (i.e., **clozapine**, **olanzapine**, **quetiapine**, and **risperidone**) and newer anticonvulsants (e.g., **sodium valproate**) in the treatment of recurrent affective disorders. This is an example of the lack of differentiation of psychiatric disorders and specificity of therapeutic efficacy.

In the maintenance phase, haloperidol and **lithium** either singly or in combination can be continued with side effects monitored. When there are depressive episodes, sodium valproate or lamotrigine ought to be considered.

Lithium Therapy

Lithium carbonate is the drug of choice in the treatment of manic psychosis. It is also effective in the maintenance or prophylaxis of bipolar illnesses. When the attacks or episodes are recurrent and close, lithium therapy should be considered. Lithium is believed to protect neurons from toxic changes in the brain during acute episodes and stress and reduce vulnerability to further attacks. **Prophylactic treatment** is long-term and safe, though it may induce complications like goitre (**hypothyroidism**), **hyperparathyroidism**, and diabetes insipidus. Long-term prophylaxis should be weighed against suicidal risk, suffering, and consequence to studies, career development, and family life. A first-year university student with an initial episode of manic-depressive psychosis would warrant lithium therapy in our competitive society.

Before lithium treatment, the following assessment is carried out. The **test panel** includes ECG, full blood count, renal screen, urine FEME, and thyroid functions. Lithium should not be given to patients with severe kidney disease, serious heart disease, or diseases with disturbance of fluid or salt balance. However, a recent meta-analysis (reported in *Lancet*, 20 Jan 2012) found that its effects on renal function and teratogenicity might be overstated. Monitoring of serum calcium levels is recommended because of parahyperthyroidism. Depending on individual differences in absorption and excretion, a daily dosage of 500–1000 mg at night or 200–400 mg twice a day can be prescribed. In our experience, the therapeutic **serum level** of lithium should be between 0.4 meq/L and 0.8 meq/L. The blood is taken 12 hours after the last dose. Blood is normally taken between 8.00 am and 8.30 am, so the patient is advised to take the last dose between 8.00 pm and 8.30 pm the night before. However, clinical response and report of side effects or complications are more important and reliable in monitoring the dosage. Periodic checks on serum lithium level, renal screen, and thyroid functions ought to be carried out.

Lithium need not be withdrawn when hypothyroidism is present. Thyroxine can be added.

During **pregnancy**, especially the first trimester, lithium should be avoided as it may cause foetal cardiac malformation. However, if a pregnant woman is on lithium treatment, it should be remembered that towards full-term, lithium is rapidly excreted. Then, at the time of delivery, the excretion rate falls abruptly back to normal. Dosages should therefore be accordingly adjusted. Lithium is best omitted during the days before and after delivery.

Recent findings suggest that termination of maintenance therapy may result in treatment resistance when the patient relapses. Thus, judgement must be carefully exercised when deciding whether to commence or terminate lithium therapy.

When lithium therapy alone is ineffective or contraindicated, carbamazepine or sodium valproate 200–400 mg twice a day may be added in combination or used as a substitute respectively. Lamotrigine can also be used for recurrent or prolonged depressive episodes. Nowadays, there is a trend to prescribe **sodium valproate** as the first-line medication in place of lithium, especially for depressive episodes. However, there have been reports that sodium valproate use is associated with **ovarian cysts**. Serious cases of drug rashes and **Steven Johnson Syndrome** have been reported in the use of **carbamazepine** and **lamotrigine.**

ECT (see earlier notes)

Treatment of "Neuroses" [Mostly Anxiety Disorders]

An Approach

It has been said that we not only need to know the bug the patient has but also the patient who has the bug. Therefore, it is desirable to find out:

Who is this patient?

Information on the patient's background and personality is essential. Certain traits and tendencies may predispose individuals to certain responses and a particular onset of the present illness. In other words, the symptoms developed could more likely be due to "personality reaction".

Why does he become ill?

The circumstances and causes that precipitate the illness should be explored in detail and in chronological sequence. Everybody has a breaking point depending on the severity of the stress experienced. However, preconceived ideas are likely to result in wrong conclusions.

What are the symptoms?

Some patients complain too much and some too little. Care should be taken to identify significant symptoms and how they develop, progress, and change. Organic diseases must always be excluded.

How are the symptoms derived?

This is something "technical" and subject to interpretation. It refers to the "defense mechanism" (e.g., denial, dissociation, displacement) employed by the unconscious to deal with anxiety-provoking stress arising intrapsychically or from the individual's own mind. Different symptoms are produced by different defense mechanisms unconsciously. All defense mechanisms serve to **repress** threatening unconscious material and prevent them from emerging into the conscious mind.

Pharmacotherapy

Anti-anxiety drugs used to consist mainly of **benzodiazepines** which act on the GABA inhibitory system. They may be divided into

short- or **long**-acting groups according to their half-life. However, recent practice appears to advocate antidepressants such as **SSRIs** over benzodiazepines. The reason is probably because patients may abuse or misuse benzodiazepines and develop dependency or addiction with dangerous consequences. As such, benzodiazepines are recommended for **acute** and **short-term** management of anxiety disorders. However, there are patients who need long-term treatment and management and do not escalate in the dosage prescribed. Judicious use and proper documentation cannot be overemphasised. The SSRIs and SNRIs act on the serotonergic and noradrenergic receptors and probably ameliorate the frequent comorbid depressive symptoms better. As different neurotransmitters and receptors are involved in the pathophysiology of anxiety disorders, it is debatable whether SSRIs and SNRIs can claim complete superiority in efficacy and safety over benzodiazepines. Paroxetine seems better indicated. Again, treatment is symptomatic and the same principles mentioned earlier apply.

Treatment of every patient should preferably be **individualised** in terms of the most suitable drug, the optimal dosage, and the frequency and timing of medication throughout the day or night to obtain best results. The **symptoms of anxiety** may be **anticipatory**, **existential**, **situational** or **sustained**, and **generalised**. Prescription should be rationalised accordingly rather than using some routine standard of, for instance, in the morning, twice a day, thrice a day, four times a day, or at night. As such, patience and cooperation from the patient are required and trial and error may be necessary. For those who are eventually prescribed pro re nata, a trial run should be carried out beforehand to test the timing of medication, efficacy, duration of action, and possible side effects.

It is always advisable to start with a lower dose (e.g., **diazepam** 2 mg, **chlordiazepoxide** 5mg, **lorazepam** 0.25 mg, **bromazepam** 1.5 mg, **clobazam** 5 mg, **dipotassium clorazepate** 5 mg) and increase according to response and requirement (rarely up to 30 mg/day for diazepam, chlordiazepoxide, clobazam, and dipotassium clorazepate; 3–4 mg/day for lorazepam; 12 mg/day for bromazepam). Treatment should aim at **maximal** if not complete **relief of symptoms**. The confidence of the patient suffering from anxiety disorders is greatly undermined by his symptoms. Therefore, when improvement occurs, medication should continue until **confidence** and **routine life** are restored. Medication should be reduced gradually without risk of relapsing symptoms.

The short-acting drugs such as lorazepam (**Ativan**) are faster in action but **dependency** is more likely to develop, especially in patients with **personality problems**. With these people, extra caution in prescribing should be exercised right from early consultations, otherwise one may end up being dictated to by them. For them, small doses of **antidepressants** (e.g., amitriptyline 10–25 mg, imipramine 25 mg) or **antipsychotics** (e.g., trifluoperazine 1–2 mg, thioridazine 10 mg) may be substituted. **Hydroxyzine**, an antihistamine 10–25 mg may also be used.

In **phobic anxiety disorders** and other anxiety disorders such as **agoraphobia** and **panic disorder** respectively, there are both **mental** and **physical** symptoms. A **combination** of imipramine 25–50 mg at night, diazepam 2–5 mg two or three times per day, and propranolol 10mg two or three times per day has been found to be effective and economical. As **different** neurotransmitters and receptors may be involved (e.g., in panic disorder), different **antidepressants** and **anti-anxiety drugs** may be indicated and trialed. Thus, **alprazolam** 0.25–1 mg two to four times per day or **moclobemide** 50–100 mg thrice per day have been found to be efficacious. As mentioned earlier, **treatment aims for complete relief of symptoms** and **restoration of confidence** and **function**. As panic attacks come with little or no warning and the symptoms pass off within minutes, pro re nata prescription has no rational basis. **Clonazepam** may be prescribed for social phobia apart from antidepressants and other benzodiazepines. For **post-traumatic stress disorder**, treatment with antidepressants and psychotherapy or cognitive behavioural therapy (EMDR) would be more appropriate. Due to HPA and hippocampal response, tianeptine may play a useful role in treatment. Prolonged medication or "medical dependence" may be unavoidable in some.

The recent anticonvulsant **pregabalin**, which decreases the release of glutamate, noradrenaline, substance P, and calcitonin, can be indicated for partial seizures, generalised anxiety disorder, neuropathic pain, and fibromyalgia. However, basic renal function tests must be done. The dosage is around 300 mg daily.

Obsessive-compulsive disorder (OCD) is related to serotonin activity or lack thereof as well as an imbalance of dopamine and acetylcholine. Therefore, drugs that are serotonergic (i.e., **clomipramine** and **SSRIs**) are employed to correct the deficiency. In addition, dopaminergic and anticholinergic drugs may also have a role in treatment.

Clinical experience shows that compulsive symptoms may be more amenable to both pharmacological and behavioural therapy combined than alone. Clomipramine would have been the preferred choice in treatment except for its intolerable strong anticholinergic (M_2, M_3) side effects. The dosage is from 25 mg to 150–200 mg at night or in divided doses. In severe cases, intravenous drips have been used. **SSRIs** (i.e., fluoxetine, fluvoxamine, paroxetine, sertraline, and escitalopram) are becoming more widely prescribed and are often used as first-line drugs and occasionally in combination. Clonazepam (long acting and with serotonergic effects) 0.5–1 mg at night may be given. Therapeutically, compulsive acts or rituals respond better to medications and behaviour therapy. Obsessional thoughts or ruminations may respond better to fluvoxamine. Sufferers of OCD are naturally distressed. However, a small number may have an underlying psychotic process and show incongruous affect. In such patients, an additional antipsychotic might help (see the OCD section on memantine and zolpidem).

Chronic depression with anxiety symptoms and **chronic anxiety** with depressive symptoms are common. **One leads to the other**, so antidepressants should be therapeutic for both. About one-sixth of affective disorders will be intractable. When there is treatment resistance, **stressors** are likely to have been persistent, so **psychosocial factors** should never be overlooked. Combined treatments do produce better results.

B. Psychological Treatment

This is particularly indicated for "neurotic" conditions. The patient should preferably **be intelligent** and **motivated**.

I. *Behaviour Therapy*

They include:
Relaxation for anxiety, tension, nervousness, phobia, and insomnia.
Desensitisation for phobias and obsessive-compulsive symptoms.
Aversion for addictive behaviours.
Flooding (in vivo) or **implosion** (in imagination) for phobias and obsessive-compulsive symptoms.
Biofeedback for control of anxiety and somatic symptoms such as pains, headaches, and tension.
Token economy for reinforcing positive behaviours in patients with chronic conditions (e.g., persons suffering from schizophrenia and mental retardation or intellectual disability).

Eye movement desensitization reprocessing (EMDR) has been used to treat PTSD. It is a technique of bilateral hemispheric stimulation and probably the dispersion or disruption of psychic materials. The visual pathway is in fact extensive, starting from the eyes, spreading into quadrants, and reaching the visual cortex in the occipital lobe. EMDR stimulation probably acts on neural connections or circuits along the long pathway to disrupt morbid patterns of response. However, the technique has evolved (e.g., tapping of body parts).

Hypnotherapy may be considered as psychotherapy under the tool or technique of **hypnosis**. The form and objective of psychotherapy depend on the formulation of the pathogenesis or psychopathology. The therapist should be a qualified professional trained to handle possible psychotic breakdowns.

Cognitive behavioural therapy is based on the hypothesis that how one feels depends on how one thinks. Symptoms are assumed to arise from faulty patterns of thought, such as generalising what is specific, jumping to conclusions, and feeling much ado about nothing, which must be systematically exposed and corrected. Sometimes, simple time management and setting of priorities help to relieve thoughts like "I am late" or "I can't meet the dateline", which can trigger anxiety or worry. Cognitive behavioural therapy is employed to treat symptoms of anxiety, depression, obsessive-compulsive disorder, and other conditions. It can be carried out in an outpatient clinic and may be combined with pharmacotherapy or psychotherapy.

The clinical psychologist is involved in the treatment and prior arrangements should be made. Several sessions may be necessary and results depend on the conscientious practice of procedures by the patients. There is some evidence that cognitive behavioural therapy is better indicated for those with vulnerable traits and predisposition to "neurotic reactions" and its efficacy is more sustainable than pharmacotherapy.

II. *Psychotherapy*

Psychotherapy, like democracy, human rights, and freedom of speech, means different things to different people. Thus, psychotherapy is practised differently by people of authority from many theoretical schools, just like how democracy, human rights, or freedom of speech is defined by people in power from many political systems. Each endeavours to convince others or impose on the lesser his views and virtues. The common factor in the different schools of psychotherapy is that the past determines the present (i.e., psychic determinism or causality).

Much has been debated on the issue of nature and nurture. There is truth to say that we are what we eat, we reap what we sow, and we are what we are downloaded with. In economics, output depends on input, and in IT language, the computer functions according to its operating system and the applications that have been installed. In psychopathology, symptoms are believed to derive from past exposure and experience. Their meaning and significance are explained according to the theory espoused. Different treatment models are thus evolved and developed.

Each school has its own hypothetical assumptions of pathogenesis and theoretical formulations of therapeutic goals based on the therapist's personal experience or observations of his own specific cultural settings, norms, and values. When uncritically practised on or prescribed for patients from different cultural backgrounds, it becomes tantamount to **downloading** on them with theoretical input and programming them for formulated output. Therapy then becomes a subtle imposition of assumptions or even colonisation of norms and desired goals extending to child development, parenting, value systems, morality, lifestyle, and interpersonal relationships. Very often, we come across patients or clients who speak like their therapists and would use the same jargon.

Nevertheless, psychotherapy may be psychoanalytical or psychodynamic, individual or group, and interpersonal. "Individual psychotherapy" in our busy clinical practice is usually **supportive** and **brief**. Patients are assisted to ventilate and gain insight. At the same time, they are given emotional support and counseling during crises.

One should be aware of the differences in **cultural norms**, **ideals**, **values**, and **lifestyles** and also be cautious of the desired outcomes hoped for. Although there are **theories** and **techniques** couched in quasi-scientific jargon, psychopathology and its management are essentially based on **psychosocial models** postulated by individuals. It is fashionable nowadays to attribute much of adult psychiatric disturbance to childhood sexual abuse. It is strange that sexual trauma is so highlighted in societies where permissiveness and promiscuity are a way of life. Much of western lifestyles, value systems, and **quality of life** are fundamentally derived from a **doctrinal subscription** to "**democracy, human rights, and freedom of speech**", which determine all enquiries and activities. Even what appears to be scientific, on closer examination, would reveal the influence of the same doctrines at work. Medical ethics are similarly derived. They are often unilaterally decided and defined as well as double standard in practice.

Therefore, we ought to be more discerning and should not borrow western definitions, theories, and practices wholesale. In our culture, patients respond better to a **more directive** and **authoritative** approach. However, there is a trend towards a **confluence of values, lifestyle, and method of parenting** that is predominant in the western world. The "**Id**" **culture** of self-gratification is already **cloning** psychiatric morbidity and the psychotherapist in our society. These trends are further prompted by the phenomenon of "**globalisation**".

C. Social Therapy

The **psychiatric nurse**, **medical social worker**, **occupational therapist**, and **case manager** play important roles in social therapy. They are pivotal in mobilising and coordinating the family and community resources. They all contribute significant therapeutic roles to the welfare and wellbeing of patients under their charge.

In the ward, the **nursing staff** ensure their personal grooming and hygiene, regular meals and medications, and their safety and sleep. Activities of daily living, recreation, and social interactions are encouraged. The **occupational therapist** provides assessment, training, and rehabilitation in social skills and work habits. Activities and treatment programmes, including art therapy, aim at integrating sensory, motor, affective, and cognitive functions. Vocational assessments and job trainings are available. Meanwhile, the **medical social worker** makes home visits, looks into the family situation and housing problems, does crisis intervention, arranges for financial assistance, and seeks job placements. The medical social worker also carries out family and marital therapy. When there are young children, more work is involved in caring for and protecting them. All efforts are concerted and coordinated to reintegrate the patient as a person back into the community. The **case manager** makes regular contact with patients, coordinates and provides feedback on their progress, and follows up to the **multidisciplinary (management) team.**

The **Agency for Integration Care** has been set up by the Ministry of Health to **oversee**, **coordinate**, and **facilitate** all efforts in integrated care. This involves **institutional, communal**, and **voluntary organisations** and **services** to enhance and integrate the long-term care sector.

Rehabilitation

Disease causes **disability**, which leads to **dependency**. There are various degrees of disability and dependency that may be **temporary** or **permanent**; **partial** or **complete**. Ideally, disease should be cured if not prevented. However, wise physicians have always said: "To cure sometimes, to care often, and to comfort always".

Mental illness is often chronic and results in chronic disability and long-term dependency. Patients need food, clothing, shelter, transport, occupation, and recreation just like anybody else. The questions then become: who should provide these needs, how are they to be provided, and where?

The aim of rehabilitation is to maximise the patient's functional capabilities and minimise his residual disabilities through proper treatment and training. The emphasis is on **recovery** and **reintegration** into the community. If the patient cannot become employable, productive, and independent, it is hoped that he can at least look after his own personal needs (e.g., eating, washing, grooming, socialising). However, some will need permanent institutional care.

Treatment and rehabilitation are inseparable, multidisciplinary effort is essential, and the family and society are also involved (e.g., their **cooperation, accommodation,** and **acceptance**). Mental patients particularly face discrimination when seeking employment. They are caught in a dilemma whether to disclose their psychiatric history when filling a job application form. Psychiatric rehabilitation is a vocation that requires **constancy** and **continuity**. Often, too little is done too late. There are also **different expectations** from the family, staff, manager, employer, and public, leading to conflict. However, with educational campaigns and manpower needs, employers have become more enlightened.

Much has been written about **institutionalisation** and its negative aspect. As a result, mental hospitals have been closed down while community care and communal living have been emphasised. However, the real force behind the decision to de-institutionalise appears to be political and administrative rather than clinical, and just like that, patients become either inmates of welfare homes or prisons or freely roaming citizens in the streets. The good intention for better quality of life in the community has suffered because of an apparent lack of resources. A solution to the dilemma had been the "day release scheme". Patients on the scheme held full time jobs outside during the day and returned to the hospital in the evening. The hostel or halfway house is midway between the hospital and community living.

It is ironic that the patient who breaks down because of stress in life should face the stress of stigma on recovery. **Stigma** is essentially due to the misconception of mental illness, fear of the unknown and uncertainty, and difficulty or inability in relating to the other person. This leads to avoidance behaviour and alienation.

It is indeed the case that **"enlightened familiarity breeds acceptance and accommodation while unenlightened familiarity breeds stigma and snubbing"** (see Nature of Stigma).

Facilities

Different **varieties** and **levels** of **facilities** should be provided for different patients, bearing in mind that **needs differ** from person to person and can **change** over time. **Case managers** are assigned to track, monitor, coordinate, and provide therapeutic continuity.

1. **Patient Education Programme**

   Patients due for discharge come together for sessions conducted by staff to educate and prepare them for life outside the hospital. Topics covered include knowledge of mental illness, importance of medication and side effects, management of anger, counseling on marriage and sex, social activities, attending job interviews, and coping with stress.

2. **Day Centres**

   These centres provide organised programmes and activities for day care, basic living skills, desirable habits, social interactions, contract work, and sheltered workshops like vocational training. Many patients become productive and find employment subsequently.

   Re-admissions and medications are significantly reduced in patients who attend the day centre regularly. These patients report sleeping better, develop confidence, and gain self-esteem. Interpersonal relationships in the family also improve.

3. **Family Education and Support**

   Sessions are held for family members to educate and counsel them regarding the nature of the patient's illness, the importance of treatment, the early detection of warning signs, and coping with the patient. The families also receive support from the staff and share their experiences with one another. Respite admission or care for the patient can be arranged.

4. **Community Psychiatry and Service**

   Community Psychiatric Nursing

   Problematic patients and families in distress can be referred to the community psychiatric nurse or team who will visit the home, make assessments (and give medication like depot in the past), arrange for admission, liaise with other services, and sort things out. When necessary, the doctor and medical social worker would be called in. Rehabilitation is offered.

Emergency Service

Emergency service sees both emergency and urgent cases and walk in cases. They may be admitted, observed, or referred for outpatient follow up. Those with long wait times for consultation may be attended by the **Home Treatment Team** during the interim period. For acute emergencies, the **Mobile Crisis Team** may be activated and mobilised. The **Community Mental Health Team** is involved in the psychosocial rehabilitation of chronic outpatients.

The **Community Engagement Team** is provided under the **Agency for Integration Care.**

Outpatient Treatment

When a patient is discharged from the ward, he is preferably followed up for a period of time in the hospital's specialist outpatient clinic or behavioural medicine clinic/community wellness clinic. Upon stabilisation, he may be referred to one of the trained general practitioners in the partnership programme for greater convenience.

Patients must be advised on the importance of **maintenance therapy** and how long they are likely to continue with treatment. **Good rapport** and **relationship** help to improve cooperation and reduce defaults. Medication must be tailored according to their requirements and daily routine. Many patients work shifts and sleep at different times. Others need to drive, handle machines, or climb heights in their jobs, and must therefore be warned of the possible dangers of side effects.

Non-compliance with medication is notorious and patients may hoard large quantities of medicines at home. Such patients must be told to return them or have their new supplies correspondingly reduced. On the other hand, there are **drug abusers** who should be blacklisted as they are known to harass and abuse doctors in busy clinics or accost other patients for their supply. They are best referred to a senior doctor in the hospital specialist outpatient clinic. Even so, other attending staff should be alerted so that when these patients pose a danger, help can be immediately summoned. The computerised appointment system has helped to prevent these patients from going to different clinics to collect medicines. If necessary, the police should be called.

Therefore, we must routinely **check** the previous dates of attendance and the treatments given. Do not repeat prescriptions blindly and do write down the date, medicines, dosages, and reasons clearly. Many, especially neurotic persons and those with personality difficulties or disorders, have become dependent on drugs because we have been too liberal in our prescriptions and failed to check or review their treatments regularly.

In a busy outpatient clinic, one may be at a loss as how to assess the patient in a few minutes. Ideally, the patient ought to be followed up by the same doctor who knows him well. Complaints of symptoms or side effects should be noted, but if they do not interfere seriously with sleep, appetite, work, and sexual life, then the patient can be said to have maintained fairly well. Therefore, routine questions on the so-called **appetites**, namely for **food, sleep, work, sex** (in its widest context), and **activity** (recreation, physical exercise, hobbies, games and social activities, addictive behaviour), that cover the whole day should be asked. Covert **psychopathology** may be revealed. Generally speaking, **work** and **performance** is an **index of wellbeing** regardless of the presence of other symptoms. For **positive mental health**, one may add the capacity for **pleasure** and **interest** as well as the presence of **energy**, **memory**, and **concentration** (i.e., **Mc PIE**) as opposed to anhedonia.

Other Subspecialist Clinics

Clinicians and other allied mental health workers with special personal interests and expertise provide more specialised clinics for various disorders in assessment and management. They include mood and anxiety disorders, OCD, insomnia, early psychosis, eating disorders, autism spectrum disorders, sexual gender dysphoria, perinatal clinic, addictive behaviour, smoking cessation, art therapy, job training, memory clinic, and neurodevelopmental assessment. More intensive psychotherapy, cognitive behavioural therapy, consultative psychopharmacology, and neurostimulation services are available.

Treatment of Insomnia

Insomnia is difficulty in falling and staying asleep. It may be **primary** or **secondary** (see Sleep Disorders), is one of the commonest complaints, and is often the presenting symptom of many underlying physical, mental, and neurological disorders. However, there are also mundane reasons such as hot weather, a noisy neighbourhood, too much excitement or overstimulation, anticipation of events, a crying baby, too much coffee or tea, physical discomfort, shift duty, and change of environment, all of which can affect one's sleep.

Management of insomnia consists of determining the **causes**, physical or psychological, and then removing them or treating them accordingly. Thus, in **psychiatric disorders**, a heavier dose of **antipsychotic**, **antidepressant** or **antimanic**, or **anti-anxiety** drugs can be given respectively for psychotic, affective, or neurotic conditions (e.g., hearing voices, fear of harm, feeling high or low in spirit, worries, palpitation, obsessional rumination).

During enquiry, different patients may have different experiences and ideas about insomnia. Some need longer hours of sleep while some can do with less. Others have fixed ideas on the number of hours required. Apart from the **quantitative** aspect of sleep, there is also the **qualitative** aspect (i.e., **non-restorative** or **refreshing sleep**). Some sleep but deny that they do while others complain that their sleep is disturbed by having too many dreams. The complaint must be properly assessed.

Patients should be asked about their physical sleeping arrangements, what time they go to bed, fall asleep, wake up, and get out of bed, what they think is the cause of their insomnia, what they do when they cannot sleep, and how they feel the next day. Organic causes such as sleep apnoea should be excluded.

In **delayed sleep phase disorder**, although we cannot force ourselves to sleep at a fixed time, we can force ourselves to wake up at a fixed time. In doing so, it is like resetting our **biological clock**. By repeatedly resetting, it is hoped that a normal biorhythm will be restored. As it is easier to delay sleep than to sleep earlier, those with **sleep-wake schedule** disorder (i.e., sleeping in the early hours of the morning and waking up around noon) can try to delay their sleep by 3 hours every day until they come back around to more normal sleeping timings.

Management

1. **Sleep Hygiene**:

   Sleep hygiene includes, for instance, a comfortable bed and environment, keeping regular hours and habits, avoidance of stimulants and stimulation, management of stress, exercise and relaxation, and a warm milk drink for night cap.

2. **Medication**

Benzodiazepines, despite the adverse publicity of addiction and dependency, are still the mainstay in the treatment of insomnia. **Judicious use** and prescription is emphasised. The shorter and faster acting ones (e.g., **triazolam, lorazepam, lormetazepam, midazolam**) are better for those having difficulty in falling asleep while the longer and slower acting ones (e.g., **flurazepam, diazepam**) are better for those with interrupted sleep. If **long-term** use is likely, drugs should be switched around, augmented by or even substituted with small doses of antipsychotics or antidepressants. In some chronic insomniacs, their socio-occupational functioning is not significantly affected. They may have to learn to accept their insomnia and not continue medication. Patients should be advised on the **rebound** phenomenon during **withdrawal** of hypnotics. Medical leave may be necessary to "rough out" treatment or withdrawal periods. Alternatively, a long-acting benzodiazepine may be introduced first, followed by withdrawal of the short-acting drug, after which the long-acting drug is tailed off.

Patients who abuse **flunitrazepam** (Roche 2) and **nimetazepam** (Erimin) are known to present in **acute psychotic** states with symptoms of hallucinations, delusional ideas, violent behaviour, disorientation, and amnesia lasting up to 2–3 days. **Suicidal** and **homicidal** behaviours may occur from such abuse. Complaints of **amnesia** are also common with the other benzodiazepines, which can affect socio-occupational functioning. **Zopiclone** (3.75–7.5 mg) and **zolpidem** (6.25–12.5 mg) are newer short-acting hypnotics with claims of inducing more normal sleep and less "hangover". However, patients on zolpidem can develop dependency and somnambulistic activities. **Hydroxyzine**, an antihistamine, has also been prescribed for insomnia. **Mirtazapine** can be an effective hypnotic and is said to preserve normal sleep structure. **Tianeptine** also seems to promote sleep when insomnia is stress-induced. Melatonin 2 mg may help with correcting the circadian rhythm.

The **timing** of medication varies with different patients and conditions. In general, 15–30 minutes before sleep is recommended. However, there are some patients (e.g., those with dementia) who respond to sedatives only hours later. It is a question of trial and error.

Treatment of Impotence and Erectile Dysfunction

Male sexual functions depend on the integrity of the cortical, spinal, peripheral, and autonomic neurological pathway as well as the hypothalamic, pituitary, adrenal, and gonadal endocrine system. There are also local anatomical or vascular factors as well as cardiorespiratory and musculoskeletal conditions. In addition, there are mental or psychic factors such as stress, anxiety, depression, and relationship strain. A conducive environment, multisensory stimulation, and voiding of the bladder and bowels may help. Organic causes may more or less be ruled out when there is presence of nocturnal penile tumescence or erection. The most common reason for poor erection and premature ejaculation is probably anxiety. In depression, libido is lowered. Psychotropic drugs with anticholinergic side effects, especially the tricyclic antidepressants, and a host of antipsychotics and other medications are also well known to cause male impotence.

In management, the principle is to reduce anxiety levels through explanation, reassurance, medication, and relaxation as well as cooperation and encouragement from the wife or partner.

Besides primary physical or mental disorders and drug-induced side effects, the libido of both males and females may be affected by their **past psychosexual development** or experience and their **relationship** with their partners. Sexual relationship and practice may reveal a whole host of psychopathology.

Phosphodiesterase Inhibitors

There are several types of **phosphodiesterases** (PDEs) distributed across nearly all of the tissues in the body and they regulate a wide variety of cellular functions. PDE3 has been used for cardio-protection and to increase insulin secretion and action. PDE4 is used in the treatment of chronic obstructive pulmonary disease, inflammatory bowel disease, autoimmune disease, and cognitive function of the brain including depression. **Sildenafil** (Viagra) and **tadalafil** (Cialis) are **PDE5** inhibitors. They are essentially vasodilators that help to improve erectile dysfunction. Due to the effects of vasodilatation, they potentiate other (organic) nitrates and can cause serious cardiovascular side effects and other medical consequences (e.g., headaches, hypotension). A thorough medical history and examination of cardiovascular disease should be carried out before prescribing such a drug. On the other hand, sildenafil has been shown to increase cardiac output and maximum workload in mountain climbers and competitive sports. It has also been used in the treatment of pulmonary hypertension and hypertension.

6 Psychiatric Services and Departments

Woodbridge Hospital and the Institute of Mental Health

Woodbridge Hospital and the **Institute of Mental Health** (WH/IMH) is the main psychiatric centre in Singapore since 1928. It provides comprehensive inpatient and outpatient services as well as training, teaching, and research in mental health. There are various departments and subspecialty divisions as well as specialist outpatient clinics, behavioural medicine clinics, and rehabilitation facilities available. The emergency service department for acute conditions and crises is open 24 hours. WH/IMH is also the centre for forensic psychiatry and remand from the Courts. There are about 2,000 beds in WH/IMH and 50,000 patient attendances for treatment annually.

In **adult (general) psychiatry**, acute patients are admitted to the short-stay wards while those who need more structured reha-bilitation or long-term custodial care are housed in the long-stay wards. Patients who are persistently disturbed, disruptive, suicidal, or violent and are compounded by personality disorders, alcohol-ism, and drug addiction are best contained in the specified wards in the forensic block. The **Adult Neurological Development Service** for autism and intellectual disability has been set up.

The **Institute of Mental Health** is a centre for teaching, training, research, and service (e.g., training of psychiatrists, clinical psychologists, and allied mental health workers), the **Early Psychosis Intervention Programme**, epidemiological studies, collaborative research projects, the **National Addiction Management Service** which comes under the new Addiction Medicine Department, psychopharmacology and drug trials, and mental health education. It organises programmes and activities such as seminars, workshops, talks, forums, and conferences on mental disorders and mental health for professionals as well as the public.

Child and Adolescent Psychiatry

The **Child Guidance Clinic** (CGC) is sited at the **Health Promotion Board**. Besides its own outpatient clinics providing consultation, treatment, and follow up, the multidisciplinary team also provides outpatient sessions at **IMH/WH** and consultative services to other ministries and institutions. Children and adolescents who are in schools or junior colleges can be referred to CGC. Otherwise, the age limit is 16 years old.

The staff of **CGC**, now known as the **Department of Child and Adolescent Psychiatry** (DCAP), also runs the inpatient **Child and Adolescent Psychiatric Unit** in WH/IMH. The child psychiatrist on call is clinically responsible and is available for consultation, but outside office hours, the medical officer on duty at WH/IMH helps to cover. Child and adolescent psychiatry service is also provided in Kandang Kerbau Hospital for Women and Children.

Children and adolescents differ from adults in that they are **growing**, **developing**, and **maturing physically**, **mentally**, **emotionally**, **socially**, and **psychosexually**. As such, they undergo changes in **defined stages**. However, growth and development do not always proceed evenly and may result in a series of chain reactions. **Variation** is to be expected and **discrepancy** is not necessarily abnormal. Like adults, they face changes and stresses in the environment as well as in themselves. The younger ones in particular manifest their problems in somatic symptoms (e.g., pains, aches), disturbance of bodily functions (e.g., feeding, sleeping, excreting), and worrisome behaviour (e.g., weepiness, fearfulness, aggression, school refusal). Often, the complaints are due to **adjustment** difficulties. In such cases, explanation, reassurance, and brief symptomatic treatment would suffice. When the complaint persists (i.e., for more than a few weeks or months except in suicidal cases), then the patient ought to be referred to the child psychiatrist for proper assessment and management.

Like adults, children and adolescents do suffer from mental disorders such as neuroses (e.g., **anxiety, depression, obsessive-compulsive disorder**), which may be grouped under **emotional disorders**, and **psychoses** (e.g., **schizophrenia** and **bipolar disorders**). The **neurodevelopmental disorders** include **autism spectrum disorders** with **Asperger's** in **DSM-5**, **specific language impairment**, dyslexia, and others. The **behaviour disorders** include opposition and defiant behaviour, antisocial or conduct behaviour, and substance abuse, which can result in disruptive behaviours, learning disabilities, and academic failure. Most of the time, it is the parents or teachers who make the complaint. It is worth reiterating that there can be a number of different diagnoses for every symptom and a number of reasons for every piece of behaviour.

There are ongoing longitudinal epidemiological studies on the **associations between mental disorders in childhood and adulthood** and the possible causes or mechanisms on the

continuities or **discontinuities** of psychopathology between childhood and adult life. Thus, the concept of **developmental psychopathology** and a **developmental perspective** have become part of mainstream inquiry. Once again, **nature** and **nurture** or **gene** and **environment interplay** is evident and important. Precursors or risk factors such as disturbance in socioemotional behaviour and motor coordination as well as abnormal suspiciousness or sensitivity may be associated with later schizophrenia. On the other hand, less than half of those with prodromal symptoms or early manifestations of the disorder will go on to develop schizophrenia, thus calling for caution in clinical intervention. Empirical evidence indicates that adolescent-onset depression is associated with strong risk of recurrence in adulthood and may be preceded by anxiety in childhood.

Over the last decade, there has been a surge in the diagnosis of **attention deficit/hyperactivity disorder** (ADHD), which has become the most frequent disorder seen at the CGC/DCAP. This may be due to changing definitions and criteria as well as better and earlier detection by informed parents and trained teachers in schools. The disorder consists of two conditions — attention deficit and hyperactivity — overlapping, is strongly influenced by genetic factors with a marked male preponderance, and can be diagnosed in early life. Two thirds of the disorder may continue into adulthood or one third of adults may not have corroborative history in childhood. The main problem seems to lie in behavioural dysregulation, executive deficits in inhibitory control and working memory, and delay aversion. Thus, **methylphenidate** probably helps through stimulation of the neuroinhibitory system or correction of hypodopaminergic effects. **ADHD** is frequently associated with oppositional or defiant behaviour and conduct problems in childhood. Follow up studies have shown that ADHD predicts later **antisocial** behaviour or disorder, but not always. Likewise, not all antisocial adults have a past history of antisocial childhood (Robins, 1966).

Comorbidities of ADHD, autism disorder, and intellectual disability are not uncommon. Childhood and adolescent conduct disorder may also be linked to substance abuse.

["Continuities and discontinuities in psychopathology between childhood and adult life" by Michael Rutter *et al.* in *Journal of Child Psychology and Psychiatry*, 2006 is recommended reading.]

In managing the child or adolescent, organic causes must always be ruled out before one looks at the family, school, neighbourhood, or peer group for clues and understanding. The child/adolescent deserves to be seen in his own right and not to be treated merely as a member of the family that is in distress. Pharmacological treatment and response may differ from adults due to brain development and a specialist should be consulted. There has been much controversy regarding suicidal risk in the treatment of young depressed patients with SSRIs (e.g., paroxetine). This is probably overexaggerated.

Childhood experience, family background, and upbringing provide insights that facilitate the prevention of disorders later in life. What is considered proper parenting should be carefully considered before advice is given. There is wisdom in cultural tradition as well as danger in modern permissiveness. We need to establish desirable mores and norms based on our own culture and shared values. **"When roles and relationships are well defined and fulfilled, stability and satisfaction in the family life can be expected."** (Stephen Fleck) In recent years, there have been "epidemics" of psychiatric disorders that, according to popular belief, are traceable to past history of childhood sexual abuse. But such memories may not be true and the definition of sexual abuse is itself controversial. Besides, childhood sexuality differs from adult sexuality. Physical contact may cause pleasure or pain but not in the adult sexual sense. Those who hold such a belief are like religious converts who, upon converting, realise their sinfulness. School bullying has also become an issue.

Response, **E**arly Intervention and **A**ssessment in **C**ommunity Mental **H**ealth (REACH), a community-based programme for students, has been set up.

Neurodevelopmental Disorders

Neurodevelopmental disorders are a group of conditions with onset during the developmental period or early childhood. Such developmental deficits may be global or specific, impair personal, social, academic, or occupational functioning, and include intellectual disability (intellectual developmental disorder) in general mental abilities, autism spectrum disorders with deficits in social communication and interaction (besides restricted repetitive patterns of behaviour, interest, or activities), and ADHD with learning disorders, communication disorders, specific learning disorders, and developmental motor disorders.

The impairments include milestone development, education attainment, language proficiency, social skills, executive functions, and independence and responsibility in activities of daily living. The more severe the deficits and impairments in mental and physical functions, the greater the likelihood of genetic and medical causative factors.

INTELLECTUAL DISABILITY (Intellectual Development Disorder)

The concepts, classifications, and approaches to management of neurodevelopmental disorders have evolved with new knowledge and understanding over the years. The old term for "**mental retardation**" was **intellectual subnormality** in **ICD-8 (1968)** irrespective of its causes. It was regarded as a state of arrested or incomplete development of mind.

When psychosis is present, the **psychotic condition** is given **priority** of classification. Similarly, where serious **personality disorder** dominates, the case should be classified accordingly.

It should be stressed that the degree of retardation according to **IQ level** is **artificial** and **unreliable**.

Direct and indirect causes of intellectual disability include:

Infections and intoxications

Trauma or physical agents

Disorders of metabolism, growth, or nutrition

Gross brain disease (post-natal)

Diseases and conditions due to (unknown) pre-natal influence

Chromosomal abnormalities

Prematurity

Major psychiatric disorders

Psychosocial (environmental) deprivation

Other and unspecified

ICD-9 (1978)

The ICD-9 defined intellectual disability as a **condition** of arrested or incomplete development of mind that is **especially characterised by subnormality of intelligence**. The coding is made on the individual's current level of **functioning** without regard to its nature or causation.

The **assessment** of **intellectual level** should be based on **whatever** information is available, including **clinical evidence**, **adaptive behaviour**, and **psychometric findings**.

IQ levels such as those based on the **Wechsler** scales are provided only as **a guide** and should **not** be applied rigidly.

Mental retardation often involves **psychiatric disturbances** and may develop as a result of physical disease or injury (i.e., acquired).

ICD-10 (1992)

The ICD-10 defined intellectual disability as a **condition** of arrested or incomplete mental development **characterised by impairment of skills** manifested during development that contribute to **overall level of intelligence** (i.e., **cognitive, language, motor**, and **social abilities**).

Retardation can occur with or without any other mental or physical disorders.

Mentally retarded individuals can experience the **full range** of mental disorders, and the **prevalence** of other mental disorders is at least **3–4 times** greater in this population than in the general population. They are also at **greater risk** of exploitation and physical or sexual abuse. **Adaptive behaviour** is always impaired, but in protected social environments where support is available, this impairment may not be at all obvious in subjects with mild mental retardation.

The presence of mental retardation does not rule out **additional diagnoses**. However, **communication difficulties** are likely to make it necessary to rely more than usual upon **objectively observable symptoms** such as, in the case of a depressive episode, psychomotor retardation, loss of appetite and weight, and sleep disturbance in order to form a diagnosis.

Diagnostic Guidelines

Intelligence is **not a unitary characteristic** but is assessed on the **basis of a large number of different and more-or-less specific skills**. Although the **general tendency** is for all of these skills to develop to a **similar level** in each individual, there can be **large discrepancies**, especially in persons who are mentally retarded.

Some may show severe impairments in one **particular area** (e.g., language) and yet exhibit a high level of competence in another particular area (e.g., in visuospatial tasks) against a background of severe mental retardation. This presents problems when determining the diagnostic category in which a retarded person should be classified.

The **assessment of intellectual level** should be based on **whatever** information is available, including **clinical findings**, **adaptive behaviour** (judged in relation to the individual's cultural background), and **psychometric performance**.

For a **definite diagnosis**, there should be a **reduced level of intellectual functioning resulting in diminished ability to adapt to the daily demands of normal social environments.**

The diagnostic category chosen should therefore be based on **global assessments of ability** and **not on any single area** of specific impairment or skill.

The **IQ levels** given are provided as **a guide** and should **not be applied rigidly** in view of the problems of **cross-cultural validity.** The categories are **arbitrary divisions** of a **complex continuum** and cannot be defined with absolute precision.

IQ should be determined from **standardised** and individually administered intelligence tests for which local cultural norms have been determined and are appropriate to the individual's level of functioning and additional specific handicapping conditions.

Mild Mental Retardation

Language development is delayed but adequate
ADL independent
Simple skills
Difficulty in academic achievement

IQ 50–69

Associated conditions such as autism, other developmental disorders, epilepsy, conduct disorders, or physical disability are found in varying proportions.

Moderate Mental Retardation

Language development is slow and limited
ADL needs supervision
Some basic skills
Limited educational achievement

IQ 35–49

Discrepant profiles of abilities are common
An **organic aetiology** can be identified in the majority

Severe Mental Retardation

Broadly similar to that of moderate mental retardation in terms of clinical picture, presence of an organic aetiology, and associated conditions.

Most people in this category suffer from a marked degree of motor impairment or other associated deficits, indicating clinically significant damage to or mal-development of the central nervous system.

IQ 20–24

Profound Mental Retardation

IQ estimated to be under 20
Severely limited in ability to understand or comply with requests or instructions

Most individuals are immobile or severely restricted in mobility, incontinent, and at most capable of only very rudimentary forms of nonverbal communication.

ADL dependent

Organic aetiology in most

Severe neurological or physical disabilities (e.g., epilepsy, visual and hearing impairments).

Pervasive developmental disorders (e.g., atypical autism).

Investigation and Management:

The more severe the disability, the more organic is the cause.

A sustained and committed **multidisciplinary** team of psychiatrists, nurses, clinical psychologists, occupational therapists, and physiotherapists is needed. Coordination and liaison with voluntary welfare organisations, community partners, and family members are essential.

The focus is on activities, exercises, language development, education, and skill training. Rehabilitation requires manpower, equipment, facilities, and space. Optimal biopsychosocial functioning is targeted. With proper and adequate management, polypharmacy due to behavioural problems, psychosis, and epileptic seizures can be minimised and quality of life may be improved.

Mental Retardation (Intellectual Disability) and Unsoundness of mind:

It has to be pointed out that the term "**unsound mind**" in the Mental Disorder and Treatment Act (1985) is **dropped** from the new Mental Health (Care and Treatment) Act (2008) and Mental Capacity Act (2008). The term "**mentally disordered (person)**" is retained (see the relevant sections).

However, "unsoundness of mind" with regards to mental retardation is still relevant in:

Penal Code
Criminal Procedure Code
Civil Law

The presence of a mental disorder (psychosis or mental retardation) is essential although, in reality, the legal criteria or tests of the issue determine the question of soundness or unsoundness of mind.

An individual's **psychometric IQ** may to some extent explain his educational achievement, optimal functioning, and social behaviour, but other factors like opportunities or privations and health status also play important roles. Hence, the notions of **"under-achieving"** and **"over-achieving"** are coined, although **one can fake low IQ but not high IQ**.

However, in **forensic issues**, the degree of mental retardation or **low IQ per se** does not determine soundness or unsoundness of mind. What matters is the individual's **capability of knowing** and **doing** regarding what is involved. The same would apply in the case of the Mental Health (Care and Treatment) Act and Mental Capacity Act.

Psychogeriatrics

Psychogeriatric patients may suffer from **different mental disorders** as well as **physical diseases**. Often, multiple conditions are present together. The common factor for both is "age" that is 65 years and above. In old age, there is ageing and failing of organs and tissues. As a result, there is **reduction** of physiological capacities and physical powers. Processes and movements are **slowed down** and **losing coordination**. **Sensory impairment** such as in vision, hearing, smelling, and posturing affects simple qualities and pleasures in life and socialising. Poor dentition affects eating. **Falls** and **fractures** are common, frequently disabling, and complicating health issues. The cliché of "golden years" is therefore misleading.

The **problems** presented are usually **multi-axial** and inter-related. Old age per se is not a problem unless there is (forced) retirement and ill health. When there is loss of employment and health without income or savings, the situation is worrying. It becomes worse when there is neither family support nor a place to stay. Loss of wellbeing, self-esteem, livelihood, and daily subsistence can lead to depression and suicide. Social agencies in ageing populations will have to plan and provide for the **retired, sickly, poor, lonely, homeless, and disabled in their progressive level of dependency and needs. Dysmnesia, depression, dementia**, and **delirium** are common (*Consultations in Geriatric Psychiatry* edited by Andrew L. H. Peh and Cheryl Loh of CGH is recommended reading).

Clinically, the principles of management are proper medications at low doses (being particularly mindful of altered metabolism, drug interactions, and risk of falls), simple procedures, safe environments, routine activities, adequate nutrition, and appropriate stimulation and hobbies, such as singing, dancing, gardening, painting, social contact, and support from caregivers. The approach should be "person-centred care". Thus, the patient's past personal and medical history, experience, nostalgia, and premorbid personality should be inquired and understood. The key to person-centredness in care is to recognise individual differences and independence and find out what most engages and stimulates them for improved quality of life.

However, more often than not, besides the clinical multidisciplinary team involved, multiple social agencies and networks need to be tapped. It is therefore important that there is a coordinator in charge to collaborate the total management. Persons in need can be referred to the **Aged Psychiatry Community Assessment and Treatment Service** in IMH.

In terms of medication, the more suitable antidepressants would be the SSRIs. Drugs with anticholinergic activity such as the tricyclic antidepressants and antipsychotics with many extra-pyramidal symptoms should be avoided. Psychotic symptoms that appear for the first time in old age may precede the onset of dementia. A low dose of quetiapine starting from 12.5 mg, olanzapine 2.5 mg, or amisulpride 50–100 mg daily may be suitable. As for dementia (Alzheimer's), the acetylcholinesterase inhibitors that are useful in the early stages of dementia include rivastigmine, galantamine, and donepezil. Cognitive functions and possibly neuropsychiatric symptoms may be ameliorated in responders. However, patients may complain of nausea, vomiting, insomnia, and diarrhoea. In addition, there may be vagal effects on the heart. **Rivastigmine** is prescribed twice a day starting from 1.5 mg and gradually increased every two weeks to 3 mg, 4.5 mg, and 6 mg. Patch is available. **Galantamine** is also prescribed twice daily starting from 4 mg and increased after 4 weeks to 8 mg and, when necessary, to 12 mg another four weeks later. **Donepezil** is given 5 mg/day and, when indicated, up to 10 mg/day after four weeks. Memory improvement takes place after 12 weeks of medication. Also available is **memantine**, an antagonist of NMDA receptors with neuroprotective functions and is thus disease-modifying. Its starting dose is 5 mg/day and gradually increased to 20 mg/day. The side effects are hallucination, dizziness, and confusion.

Alcoholism and Treatment

Alcohol is a daily diet and a potential drug to millions of people. The making and selling of alcohol is big business while excessive drinking has brought about suffering and disruption to the problem drinker and others around him. Alcohol in suitable amounts is enlivening and pleasurable. It acts by stimulating the release of noradrenaline, dopamine, and the endogenous opioids. The latter two neurotransmitters are involved in the reinforcing actions of most drugs of abuse (Nutt). People also take alcohol to reduce anxiety. Its anxiolytic action occurs through increasing inhibition of the GABA system and decreasing excitation of the glutamate system (particularly N-methyl-D-aspartate or NMDA receptors). However, at higher concentrations of increasing toxic proportions, ataxia, amnesia, and asphyxiation can occur. During withdrawal, there is a combination of decreased central inhibition and increased excitation. Symptoms of increased sympathetic activity from noradrenergic overdrive are obvious. The effects of alcohol on the brain are very complex as it interacts with both the excitatory and inhibitory systems. Prolonged and heavy drinking can lead to brain damage with symptoms of seizures, blackouts (amnesia), and dementia.

Alcoholism is a general term for conditions and disorders related to excessive intake of alcohol and its dependence. According to Cloninger and colleagues, **type 2 early-onset** alcoholics are low in brain serotonin, poor in impulse control, and associated with psychopathy or criminality, whereas **type 1 late-onset** alcoholics have high levels of serotonin function with personality traits involving high harm avoidance and anxiety. The effects of alcohol-induced **medical diseases** are well known. Apart from gastritis or ulcer, haematemesis, avitaminosis, malnutrition, liver/pancreas disease, cardiomyopathy, and sexual dysfunction, alcohol also affects the cortex, cerebellum, pons, midbrain, brainstem, spinal cord, and cranial or peripheral nerves.

Mental or **neuropsychiatric disorders** include acute and chronic brain syndromes, such as **delirium tremens** and **dementing symptoms**, respectively. **Pathological intoxication** with aggressive and violent outbursts can occur in susceptible individuals. Morning drinking to reduce "morning shakes" from mild withdrawal is evidence of alcoholism. **Auditory hallucinosis** may or may not be due to withdrawal. In **Korsakov's** psychosis, the outstanding symptoms are amnesia and confabulation. Finally, another important complication of alcoholism is **morbid jealousy**, which may be preceded by **low libido** and symptoms of **impotence** in male drinkers. This delusional disorder can lead to grave consequences including homicidal behaviour and become a **forensic** problem.

Chronic alcoholism not only causes **physical** diseases and **mental** disorders but also brings about a host of **social** problems. It is frequently associated with symptoms of insomnia, anxiety, and **affective disorders**. Excessive drinking during **pregnancy** may affect foetal development. Marital and family life, work performance and employment, income and financial state, social relationships, and public behaviour (e.g., driving accidents, violence) are all affected. Thus, the alcoholic not only creates problems for himself but also for his family and society as a whole. The causes of alcoholism are **multifactorial** and the management is truly **multidisciplinary**.

Motivation for treatment and recovery is of utmost importance. The individual must be prepared to follow a structured programme or regime rigorously and religiously. **Detoxification** can be carried out on an outpatient basis. Acute medical treatment includes correction of fluid balance and nutritional deficiency (i.e., vitamins B1 and B12, folic acid) and sedation with

benzodiazepines and/or **antipsychotics** during withdrawal periods. Relapse prevention is an uphill and unending task. **Medications** depend on an understanding and hypotheses of symptoms production. For aversion therapy, **disulfiram** has been used, but not without risk as it blocks oxidation of alcohol and leads to accumulation of acetaldehyde with complaints of flushing, headache, choking sensations, rapid pulse, and feelings of anxiety. The opioid receptor antagonists (i.e., **naloxone** and **naltrexone**) are effective in reducing the reinforcing actions of alcohol. Like alcohol, **acamprosate** stimulates GABAergic inhibition and suppresses glutaminergic excitation, so in this "simulative" way, alcoholics conditioned with acamprosate may be less activated by the cues of sights, smells, and sounds that have been associated with alcohol use (Nutt). As $5HT_{1A}$, $5HT_2$, and $5HT_3$ receptors are implicated in various symptoms and behaviours of alcoholism, antidepressants (both agonists and antagonists) have a role in treatment.

Psychosocial treatment in terms of understanding, empathy, counselling, and support is most important. Regular group sessions are held for alcoholics and also separately for their families. Self-help groups like **alcoholics' anonymous** provide identification and fellowship and foster collective effort in maintaining sobriety. The scale of progress and success in the treatment of alcoholism is measured in small steps and from day to day. Relapses from **abstinence** are common.

Addiction

An Overview

"Addiction" is mainly used to refer to dependency on substance use via oral ingestion, inhalation, or intramuscular and intravenous routes. The "substance" is generally a psychoactive drug that has been medically prescribed, misused, or abused. This concept of dependency that is apparently driven by a compulsive need and craving behaviour for drugs, beverages, and food has been extended to non-substance appetites such as sex, gambling, computer games, internet surfing, and other activities (e.g., repeated offence).

The urge for the substance or activity is to derive comfort, pleasure, and stimulation or to suppress discomfort and distress from its withdrawal. The first experience of the substance or activity may be voluntary or involuntary and the outcome may be positive or negative depending on the individual and the circumstance. What follows depends on the multiplicity of predisposing, precipitating, and propagating factors, which can be biological, psychological, social, and spiritual. For many perhaps, it is just a one-off curiosity or experiment and if some do continue, they do so with voluntary control over themselves and their experience. For others, it may be a case of "love at first try", after which they pursue involuntary control. For some, the first try may be an unpleasant experience, but for various reasons they may persevere voluntarily and do experience comfort and pleasure eventually — an "acquired taste", so to speak. Subsequently, tolerance and dependency develop and voluntary control is lost. These people then continue involuntarily and are enslaved without deriving any enjoyment. Often, more than one substance and/or activity are involved or combined.

Psychologically, the path to addiction or dependency may begin with the cognitive intent to experience. However, it may be associated with the individual's affective state or symptomatic of underlying anxiety or depression, which may perpetuate the substance use or activity. The mind and heart go hand in hand. As the course progresses, the cognitive will or resistance weakens and gives in to physiological response and emotional distress. Attempts at control and abstinence fail when cognition and affect exposed to environmental cues and personal experiential tension are overwhelmed and the past convergent memory set of experience and habit is released.

Psychological and physiological processes normally react, change, and adapt. However, when adaptation breaks down, stereotyped responses emerge. It could be said that when habits become a reflex, the default automatic system kicks in. The habit of addiction perpetuated by this default and automatic drive system does not seem to serve any purpose except to go in circles. It is not rewarded with pleasure or stimulation and is indulged in despite suffering and punishment.

Due to similar compulsive features, habits, and impulse control disorders, obsessive-compulsive disorder, tics, Tourette's syndrome, bulimia, and so on have been linked in overlapping psychopathology. Broadly, the neurological systems comprising the inhibitory GABA system, the excitatory glutamate system, the serotoninergic (impulse control) system, the stimulating opioid/endorphin system, and the dopaminergic system as well as their interplay appear to be involved in pathophysiology. The latter two neurotransmitters are said to be involved in the reinforcing actions of most drugs of abuse, and they form the basis for rational psychopharmacological interventions.

Approach to Management

The substance use disorders, habits (addictive), and impulse control disorders are a highly heterogeneous and complex set of disorders. The approach should be holistic and the management should be individualised and eclectic. Each individual ought to be evaluated separately and understood in terms of his/her predisposing, precipitating, and propagating/perpetuating factors. When his/

her biological, psychological, social, and spiritual attributes are factored in, there are multiple combinations and permutations of interrelations, interactions, and integrations or disintegrations. The aims are to reduce aggravating factors in areas identified and to strengthen or restore cognitive and affective control.

For consultation, it is also necessary to determine the stage of the course of addiction where the problem presents. Voluntary control should not be allowed to slide into involuntary control and pleasure should be restrained before giving way to distress. The problem is best "**nipped in the bud**" through education and avoidance or prevention of temptation when potential risks exist, such as in certain subcultures or lifestyles, peer influence or pressure, occupational hazards, pathological family history, and vulnerable personality profiles. A Hong Kong study shows that people with **unfounded confidence in indulging** (e.g., "I won't get addicted", "I will win this round") and **desire for quick gratification** (e.g., effect or result is experienced with little delay) are the very ones who are most likely to get addicted. In psychological management, the general principles are to reward and reinforce desirable positive responses or deter and "punish" undesirable negative responses. Policy and legislation, manipulation of the physical and social environment, and group support are needed.

The medical model is based on an understanding or belief of the neurotransmitters and receptors (and their interplay) that are implicated in addiction and addictive behaviour. The principles involve employing appropriate drugs to block negative impulses and behaviour, canceling or negating the reinforcing effects of habits, inducing aversion responses to habits, alleviating underlying symptoms of distress or psychopathology, and treating or preventing symptoms of intoxication or withdrawal. On the other hand, a latest Hong Kong study indicates that more than half of problem gamblers also suffer from one or more psychiatric disorders.

Different strategies are advocated in different treatment programmes. Besides psychopharmacological intervention, there are abstinence-oriented treatments, replacement therapies, and controlled substance use and habit approaches. Essentially, patients must be matched to treatments and treatments must be matched to the course of the disorder.

The **Substance Abuse and Mental Health Services Administration** (SAMHSA), published online on 22 December 2011, states:

Study Highlights

- SAMHSA defines "recovery" from mental disorders and substance use disorders as a process of change through which **individuals** improve their health and wellness, live a self-directed life, and strive to reach their full potential.
- The Recovery Support Strategic Initiative has identified four major dimensions that support a life in recovery: **health, home, purpose, and community.**
- **Health** is defined as overcoming or managing the disease and living in a way that promotes physical and emotional health.
- **Home** is defined as a stable and safe place to live.
- **Purpose** refers to meaningful daily activities, such as work, school, volunteering, family caregiving, or creative pursuits, accompanied by the independence, income, and resources to participate in society.
- **Community** refers to relationships and social networks offering support, friendship, love, and hope.
- Guiding principles of recovery include the following:

  o Recovery stems from **hope**, which is internalised and can be encouraged by peers, families, providers, allies, and others.

o   Recovery is **person driven**, based on self-determination, self-direction, definition of patients' own life goals, and design of their own unique path(s) to attain these goals. Optimising patient autonomy and independence empowers patients and gives them the resources to make informed decisions, begin recovery, build on their strengths, and gain or regain control of their lives.

o   Recovery occurs via **many pathways**, based on each individual's unique needs, strengths, preferences, goals, culture, backgrounds, and trauma experiences. Pathways may include professional clinical treatment; medications; support of family, school, and peers; faith-based approaches; and abstinence for those with substance use disorders.

o   Recovery is **holistic**, involving mind, body, spirit, and community, and integrating self-care practices, family, housing, employment, education, clinical treatment, faith, spirituality, creativity, social networks, transportation, and community participation.

o   Peers and allies **support** recovery through mutual support and mutual aid groups, as do professionals by providing clinical treatment and other services.

o   **Relationship** and **social networks** support recovery by allowing the patient to leave behind unhealthy and/or unfulfilling life roles and to engage in new roles, such as a partner, caregiver, friend, student, or employee.

o   Recovery is **culturally based and influenced**, with values, traditions, and beliefs determining a person's journey and unique pathway to recovery. Services should be culturally grounded and personalised.

o   Addressing **trauma** — including physical or sexual abuse, domestic violence, war, and disaster — supports recovery, as these forms of trauma often precede or are associated with alcohol and drug use, mental health problems, and related issues.

o Recovery **involves** individual, family, and community strengths; and responsibility.

o Recovery is based on **respect** and requires protecting patient rights and eliminating discrimination. All concerned should acknowledge that taking steps towards recovery may require great courage. Self-acceptance and a positive sense of identity promote recovery.

Under the National Addictions Management Service, a separate **Clinic C** has been set up in IMH to cater for this group of patients.

Forensic Psychiatry

Abnormal offenders remanded by the **court** for **psychiatric assessment** and **report** are admitted to the forensic psychiatry wards in WH. They may be found fit or unfit to plead and of sound or unsound mind at the time of the commission of the offence. Those who are unfit and/or unsound will be detained and reviewed regularly by the Visitors' Board, which will propose appropriate recommendations to the Minister for Law.

The forensic wards also look after patients who are **refractory**, **violent**, and **dangerous**.

Special procedures are laid down for forensic patients with medical or surgical emergencies. The first line of action is to refer them to Changi Prison Hospital. However, if the condition cannot be handled at Changi Prison Hospital, then the patient should be sent to Changi General Hospital (or another designated hospital). If specialised attention is required, the patient should be referred to the appropriate hospital. Full instructions regarding referrals are kept in each forensic ward. All forensic patients need **police escorts** when leaving the ward.

Psychological Medicine Unit(s)

There are Departments of Psychological Medicine or Psychiatric Units in virtually all general hospitals in Singapore. Specifically, these are the National University Hospital, Singapore General Hospital, Tan Tock Seng Hospital, Changi General Hospital, Khoo Teck Puat General Hospital, Ng Teng Fong General Hospital, Kandang Kerbau Women's and Children's Hospital, and Seng Kang General Hospital. They treat patients with general psychiatric disorders in adults and some in children as well. Not all provide inpatient beds. Besides providing liaison psychiatry, some have subspecialties in eating and sleep disorders or even in addiction medicine and may run their own inpatient, outpatient, and rehabilitation services. However, patients who are too disturbed, violent, or suicidal and show absconding tendencies are referred to WH/IMH for inpatient management. Patients with forensic issues are also referred.

Psychiatric Treatment in Pregnancy or During the Reproductive Period

(Dr. Helen Chen *et al*, KKH)
Generally speaking, this approach to treatment can only be a **guideline** based on **anecdotal** cases and **retrospective** studies since **ethics** do not permit clinical drug trials risking embryonic development and foetal wellbeing.

The reproductive period of female patients may be divided into **preconception, pregnancy**, and **postpartum**. As a guide, due to **potential toxicity** to the mother and **risk of teratogenicity** to the embryo or foetus, medication is **best avoided** if possible, especially when there is a plan to have a baby (i.e., before conception and during the first trimester of pregnancy, which is the period of organogenesis). However, management decisions must be precluded by a **proper and complete history**. This includes the patient's **past psychiatric history** and the **family's history of mental disorders**. If the patient has had one or more prior episodes of mental illness, the **nature**, **severity**, and **frequency** of the disorder ought to be enquired. It is also important to assess her **marital status**, **relationship(s)**, and the **family** and **social support** available, which will help in planning the management and therapeutic alliances.

As much is still unknown or uncertain, the patient should be told clearly the **potential risks** and **benefits** of medications so that she and her partner or family can make **informed treatment decisions**, all of which must be **properly documented.**

Based on what is known so far, the various classes of drugs from anecdotal experiences are suggested as follows:

Antidepressants

On 8 July 2015, *BMJ* reported in a study of 28,000 women that there was no increased risk of birth defects from **citalopram** and **sertraline**. However, it confirmed two previously reported birth defects associated with **fluoxetine** (i.e., heart wall defects and craniosyntosis) and five previously reported birth defects associated with **paroxetine** (i.e., cardiovascular defects and anencephaly). Although this is 2 to 3.5 times more frequent among infants of women taking fluoxetine and paroxetine early in pregnancy, researchers noted that absolute risk was low.

In the second trimester, barring side effects, **TCAs** may be preferred to **SSRIs** which risk pulmonary hypertension in the newborn. However, in the first trimester, because the risks of SSRIs are a little more understood, informed consent and decision may make their use more acceptable relative to TCAs, which remain less examined to date. Specific drugs and risk of specific birth defects ought to be noted and reported.

Anxiolytics (i.e. benzodiazepines)

Anti-anxiety medicines may cause floppy baby syndrome and sedation.

Antipsychotics

First-generation antipsychotics like trifluoperazine and haloperidol may be preferred and there is good evidence suggesting that olanzapine is relatively safe despite its metabolic side effects. However, quetiapine and risperidone are also prescribed by local clinicians.

Mood stabilisers and anticonvulsants

Mood stabilisers and anticonvulsants are used mainly in bipolar disorders and may be associated with ovarian cysts.

Lithium may cause cardiac abnormalities to the early foetus and toxicity to the mother towards the time of delivery. Close monitoring and titration are necessary during the last two weeks of the third trimester and during peuperium. Peripartum lithium therapy should only be done by trained and experienced specialists (see also the section on lithium therapy).

Sodium valproate and **carbamazepine** may cause neural tube malformation and are also associated with low IQ. Children exposed in utero to **valproate** are at heightened risk of serious developmental disorders (up to 30–40% of cases experience delays in their early development such as talking and/or walking, have low intellectual abilities, poor language skills, and memory problems) and/or congenital malformations (in approximately 10% of cases). The risk of abnormal pregnancy outcomes is dose dependent.

Lamotrigine appears to be the safer drug, though it may cause cleft palates. Adverse effects (e.g., rashes, bullous skin lesions, Steven Johnson Syndrome) must be looked out for.

ECT

In severe and emergency situations, ECT should be considered. Its use in pregnancy is safe and does not cause uterine contractions, and results may be remarkable.

Peuperal psychosis refers to a psychotic episode during peuperium and occurs in about 1:1000 of pregnancy cases. The clinical presentation may be **pleomorphic** with a **mixture** of symptoms not unlike schizophrenia, bipolar disorder, and organic psychosis combined. It may resolve well with antipsychotics or become prolonged and differentiate into more obvious psychotic depression, bipolar disorder, or schizophrenia and **recur** later in life. Family history may offer clues. Maintenance treatment must be considered in those with recurrent episodes and positive family history of severe mental illness. For some women who present early for treatment and have minimal risks, short-term treatment can be sufficient and indeed beneficial.

Breastfeeding is contraindicated in mothers on lithium therapy, but as suggested from evidence from nursing mothers with epilepsy, sodium valproate and carbamazepine are not incompatible. There is limited evidence about lamotrigine safety in lactation. Mothers should be supported in their decision to breastfeed as the benefits are significant. Treatment can be modified to support this (e.g., using minimum effective doses in divided dosing and possibly after feeding or expression). The condition of the baby should be assessed.

Overall Management

In principle, when the decision to treat is reached, the drug used should commence with **low doses** and increase only gradually.

Not only should medication be closely supervised and monitored, but **psychosocial support** should also be ensured and provided. Indeed, **psychological therapy** and support should remain the **first-line** and **mainstay interventions** whilst medication is considered for those with moderate to severe depression. The patient and family should also be given psycho-education and social support when long-term follow up is expected of the mental disorder that is suffered.

In addition, the patient's **fitness** and **worthiness to motherhood** should be **reassured** and **encouraged**. As far as possible, mother and baby should not be separated so as to allow confidence and bonding to develop.

Military Psychiatry

[Drs. Christopher Cheok and Jared Ng — Chapter 28, Essential Guide to Psychiatry, 2014]

In Singapore, male citizens who are 18 years of age are liable for enlistment into the **Singapore Armed Forces** (SAF) for two years of **national service** (NS). Pre-enlistment screenings on fitness to serve are carried out before each intake. Upon successful completion of NS, which is known as the **operationally ready date**, he is further liable for periodic callups of short-term **reservist** exercise. Academic, social, occupational, and family life will be delayed or disrupted. On the other hand, disruption of or exemption from national service will be a disadvantage when seeking employment in future. The career regular personnel can be on contract until 45–50 years old. There are neither pension nor medical benefits thereafter.

SAF is a **defence force** whose mission is to protect Singapore, a small island city-state without natural resources other than its manpower. Our survival depends on having a strong defence in a peaceful and stable regional environment as well as an open and globalised economy. The twin pillars of Singapore's defence policy are **deterrence** and **diplomacy**, which undergirds the role and duty of NS.

Broadly, the different workgroups in the SAF and Military Culture consist of:

a. Uniformed soldiers (NSF)
b. Defence Executive Officers
c. Defence Contractors

Their physical employment status, which ranges from A to F, is their medical classification in terms of fitness and determines their vocational placement. Peer influence in late adolescents and young adults plays an important role in influencing satisfactory adjustment or developing psychopathology and social issues.

Factors for Poor Mental Health leading to Poor Work Performance:

a. Education Attainment — lower level, higher risk
b. Home Environment — parental divorce, history of suicide, death, mental illness, criminality, financial problems, and being away for long periods of time as a child
c. Marrying young and being a father while serving as a NSF — lower education and income, unplanned pregnancy

Importance of Fulfilling Basic Needs in Life:

Our physiological and psychological needs include safety, love, belonging, self-esteem, and actualisation. To manage at-risk groups, it is necessary to note their personality, coping styles, and belief systems as well as the abovementioned risk factors:

a. Psychological origins of the NSF's attitudes towards life and NS and his unmet needs.
b. Motivation through care for his dignity and respect.
c. Patience to overcome long-term accumulated needs and sufferings.
d. Commander's responsibility to modify the social environment and change work responsibilities and place of work.

Overview of Psychological Problems faced by regulars:

1. Young regulars
Common issues affecting young regulars include:
a) Adapting to military training courses, which can separate the soldier from his family for significant periods of time, especially for trainees in the navy.
b) Discovering that they do not like a military career and yet are still bonded to the job.
c) Adapting to military culture.
d) Long hours that may be irregular and being put on standby for missions.

2. Mid-career regulars
Common issues affecting mid-career regulars include:
a) A competitive and stressful work environment with missed opportunities for advancement or promotion.
b) Marital problems due to long working hours and extramarital affairs by either partner.
c) Overseas deployments for training or military operations.
d) Deciding whether to extend their military career.
e) Increasing complexity and responsibilities from assigned jobs.

f) Financial worries such as providing for one's family due to one's current phase of life.

3. **End-career regulars**

Common issues affecting end-career regulars include:

a) Deciding when and how to transit into retirement or a second career.

b) Anxiety over choice of second career beyond the military career.

c) Anxiety over one's ability to adapt to a non-military work environment.

d) Anxiety over loss of income upon retirement or in the second career.

e) Marital problems.

Common Mental Illnesses affecting NSFs:

a. **Adjustment disorder (most common during the first 6 months)**

b. **Psychosis and early presentation**

c. **ADHD**

d. **OCD**

e. **Mood disorders and depression**

f. **Addictions (e.g., internet, gaming, gambling, drug abuse)**

g. **Autism and pervasive developmental disorders**

h. **Self-harm**

There are psychiatrists, medical specialists, psychologists, counselors, social workers, and medical orderlies in SAF providing basic services in their respective centres. However, more complex, acute, and severe psychiatric cases are referred to IMH/WH for inpatient or more comprehensive management.

There are some who serve their national service in the **Singapore Police Force** or **Singapore Civil Defence Force**.

They come under their own separate administrations and management.

Nature of Stigma

Meanings/Concepts of Stigma:
The meanings and concepts of stigma include alienation, blemish, contamination, contempt, condemnation, disgrace, disdain, derision, despisal, discrimination, fear, and shame.

Origins of Stigma:
The origins of stigma include a sense of superiority and self-righteousness, being set apart and aloft, ignorance, misconception or misunderstanding, prejudice, fear of the unknown, uncertainty, and unpredictability.

Subjects or Contexts of Stigma:
Stigma has existed since ancient times. It is present in many cultures and situations and for many individuals in varying degrees ranging from mild and subtle to strong and obvious. It may occur in primitive and underdeveloped societies or in ethnic groups with distinct social classes and castes. It may also be due to cultural and religious customs and taboos. For instance, one may be stigmatised when unmarried past a certain age, for being in a mixed marriage, for being an unwed mother, when born out of wedlock, for being divorced, or when caught committing adultery.

Stigmatization of superstition may cause individuals who are superstitious to be looked down on as being ignorant. In lifestyle and occupation, it may apply to poverty, sex workers, menial and lowly jobs, unemployment, illegal activities, prisoners, and ex-convicts. In medical contexts, it is well known to apply to sufferers of mental disorders or medical illnesses. It commonly involves individuals with sexually transmitted diseases, HIV/AIDS, cancer, dementia, intellectual disabilities or mental retardation, disfigurement, and (more so in the past) sexual gender dysphoria or orientation, leprosy, and tuberculosis, including even the personnel or professionals who look after them. Changes in what people stigmatise are due to better understanding, efficacious treatment, and hope of recovery unlike attitudes in the past that view these conditions as incurable like a death sentence.

Core issue — due to "Not knowing how to relate to the other person"

The core issue of stigma in mental illness or disorder appears to be that of "**not knowing how to relate to the other person**" due to factors such as discrimination, ignorance, fear, lack of exposure and contact, or misconceived influence from others. This is particularly experienced by **psychosis** sufferers as there is a **breakdown** in **conformity** of appearance and behaviour **with the community**, a **breakdown** in **interpersonal communication** because of incoherent or irrational and irrelevant thought and speech, and a **breakdown** in **control** when they act out their psychotic experience in a frightening or threatening manner that cannot be understood or predicted. As a result, there is uneasiness, discomfort, fear, and being at a loss as to what to do and how to respond to the person, leading to avoidance.

Thus, stigma occurs when there is breakdown in conformity (with the community), breakdown in communication (interpersonally), and breakdown in control (of the individual). Relationships become distant and alienated or discriminated and even condemned. Due to ignorance, misconception, prejudice, and misgivings or fear of the unknown, uncertainty, and unpredictability, this stigma is **extended to other mental disorders** such as anxiety, depression, and obsessive-compulsive symptoms, which are **common** and **prevalent** and may affect **anyone**. Stigma perpetuates in a vicious cycle when symptoms are concealed, consultation is avoided, or treatment is noncompliant. But when one is well informed of the nature of mental illness and trained, engaged, and experienced in managing or understanding them, what is stigmatising then wears away.

There is a saying that "**familiarity breeds contempt**". It is actually **unenlightened** familiarity that breeds stigma and snubbing. **Enlightened** familiarity breeds acceptance and accommodation. Families and mental health professionals show that relationships can develop and stigma can be reduced. "Sufferers" can lead by example and demonstrate that recovery and reintegration are possible and provide peer support.

It should be kept in mind that the earlier the assessment, the earlier the treatment, the earlier the recovery, the earlier avoidance of stigma. Sustained treatment leads to sustained recovery and a reduction in relapses and impairment.

Comparison of Mental Disorders and Medical Disabilities

The physically disabled are viewed with great sympathy and understandably so. There are braille and white sticks for the blind and sign language and speech therapy for the deaf and mute. There are many voluntary organisations and lobby groups advancing their rights and interests. Jobs are created or reserved for them. Specially modified cars, reserved parking lots, wheelchairs, ramps, lifts in buildings, user-friendly toilets, public transport with special facilities, and easier access to places of interest are provided. However, the mentally disabled are avoided, ignored, or even rejected. The blind cannot be expected to see, the deaf cannot be expected to hear, and paraplegics cannot be expected to walk like normal people, but people bend backwards to help and accommodate them and even invent robotics and prostheses to rehabilitate them. Thus, the public and sometimes our own rehabilitation programmes expect if not demand that the mentally disordered behave and function like ordinary people. But people with severe volitional and cognitive impairments are dysfunctional, like the "psychic tetraplegic" or the computer that hangs. Indiscriminate overenthusiasm can be stressful and counterproductive.

The **consequences of stigma** in mental illness or disorder include covering up, secrecy, avoidance, alienation, discrimination in employment, noncompliance in treatment, and suffering with loss in productivity and dependency.

Management:
Continual proper education, appropriate exposure, engagement, or experience, and sustained campaigns for the public and volunteers are necessary. There must also be "enlightened familiarity" so that people can relate to one another with compassion, acceptance, and accommodation.

Strategic Goals:
Subjective Perceptions: There must be understanding, acceptance/accommodation, support, compassion, and hope

Objective Targets: There must be public campaigns/ education, social reform, removal of questions pertaining to mental illness in job applications, medical research/treatment, improved prognosis/hope of recovery, economic opportunities, political legislation

Promoting Mental Health

It is said that there is **no healthy person** (whether physical, psychological, or social) **without a healthy environment**. Hence, there is an active balance between the health of individuals and the environment.

Apart from mental disorders of known biological or organic causes, the **majority** of mental disorders can be said to be **induced by stress or stressors in life**. As such, both predisposed **intrinsic** factors of individual vulnerabilities and **extrinsic** factors of environmental pressures underlie mental disorder.

So far, mental health programmes and strategies **focus** mainly on suffering individuals or casualties. Management emphasises early detection, early treatment (e.g., coping with stress), providing hotlines and community and welfare services, medication, psychotherapy, and lifestyle changes. However, if **prevention is better than cure**, then there should be an increased **focus** on or recognition of the **unhealthy environment**, which is often the **causative** factor or stressor. Stress management ought to involve **employers** (including managers, executives, and supervisors), the **government** and its policy enforcements, and **public** perceptions and attitudes.

With preoccupation on **economic growth**, there is constant emphasis on competition, restructuring, skill upgrading, productivity, consumerism, and materialism. Although stress is unavoidable to ensure survival, it is not always necessary. To reduce mental health casualties, there needs to be a paradigm shift in the responsibility of the environment and system (in its management) in order to reduce **unnecessary stress** due to selfishness, greed, and incompetency.

It should also be kept in mind that for every solution decided, a price must be paid by someone, somewhere, sometime. It takes insight and effort to achieve a more humane balance that minimises fall out.

Miscellaneous

Certification of Deaths

Non forensic deaths of known causes in Woodbridge Hospital can be certified by the doctor on duty. Forensic deaths of unknown causes are Coroner's cases and special forms must be filled. It should be noted that certification of death is not the same as certi-fication of the cause of death, which is the Coroner's job.

Voluntary Welfare Organisations

Apart from government psychiatric services, voluntary organ-isations play important roles in providing complementary or supplementary community services. The relevant services or facil-ities include care and counselling centres, social service centres, the New Horizon Centre for Alzheimer's disease, day care and family service centres, welfare services and homes, homes for the elderly, and halfway houses. Most of these facilities are run by vol-untary organisations or are associated with religious groups. Oth-ers include the Singapore Association for Mental Health, Samar-itans of Singapore, Movement for the Intellectually Disabled, Alcoholics Anonymous, Singapore Anti-Narcotic Association, and Singapore Anglican Community Services, which runs the Hougang and Simei Care Centres for rehabilitation and services for autistic patients.

Medical social workers will be able to advise on how to approach these agencies for help. A directory of social services in Singapore is available.

The Ministry of Health has set up the **Agency for Integration Care** to oversee, coordinate, and facilitate all efforts in integrated care. This involves institutional, communal, and voluntary organisations and services to enhance and integrate the long-term care sector.

7 Law and Psychiatry

Law is concerned with the protection of individuals and properties in society and defines what crime is. As such, what was crime yesterday may not be crime today and what is crime today may not be crime tomorrow, each according to the law of the land.

Psychiatry is the branch of medicine that diagnoses and treats mental disorders. It concerns doctor-patient relationships and ethics.

Forensic psychiatry is the application of psychiatry in legal processes. In general, it involves assessment of issues regarding credibility (e.g., as witness), culpability (e.g., in crime), competency (e.g., when making a will or contract), compensation (e.g., to injury), and custody (e.g., of a child). (**Slovenko**)

Terminology and Concepts

Madness	—	lay idea
Insanity/Lunacy	—	legal concept (unsoundness of mind)
Psychosis	—	medical term
Mental Disorder	—	generic term for all psychiatric conditions

Mental Illness	—	traditionally refers to psychosis and neurosis
Mental Disease	—	old term for psychosis/insanity
Disease of the Mind	—	legal term

Theories and Models of Mental Disorders

Biological/Medical Concept	—	Pathological abnormality
Social/Cultural Concept	—	Statistical deviation
Psychological/Behavioural Concept	—	Developmental impairment
Spiritual/Religious Concept	—	Supernatural visitation

More often than not, there is an interplay and overlapping of factors.

Forensic Psychiatry in:

A. Penal Code

Concept of Responsibility

Man is presumed to be a free agent who acts according to his intentions. This presumption forms the basis of every criminal code and system of punishment. However, some are less responsible than others. "Excuses" from responsibility may include young age, mistakes, accidents, provocation, duress, and insanity. There is also a tendency by some to medicalise transgressions (e.g., sin is due to sadness or "he is so bad, he must be mad").

Criminal responsibility is essentially a legal matter to be determined by the jury. In Singapore, the judge decides as the jury system has been abolished.

Actus Reus

An illegal act or omission has occurred and has been carried out by an identified person. In addition, the act or omission must cause the offending consequences.

Mens Rea

This refers to the presence of **intent** (or guilty mind) specific to the particular offence. The mental state in question concerns largely cognitive and not emotional aspects.

Theoretically, when there is no intent, there is no crime. However, in practice, intent is presumed when there is an offence. In **automatism**, certain acts are carried out but without awareness. This would imply absence of intent and, therefore, absence of criminal responsibility.

In reality, however, legal outcomes depend on the underlying causes of non-awareness. If the cause is not one of insanity, then it leads to acquittal. However, if the cause is one of insanity and/or is inherent in nature, then the verdict is unsoundness of mind. Epilepsy and somnambulism are examples of "disease of the mind" and individuals with such conditions have been judged as legally insane because of the inherent danger of recurrence.

McNaughton Rules

"To establish a defence on ground of insanity it must be clearly proven that at the time of the committing of the act, the accused was labouring under such a defect of reason from disease of the mind as not to know the nature and quality of the act or if he did know it that he did not know he was doing what was wrong."

The **defect of reason** refers to cognitive impairment. In **"disease of the mind"**, the mind is seen in the ordinary sense of mental faculties of reason, memory, and understanding. Thus, if these faculties are impaired, disease of the mind is present and it matters not whether the aetiology of the impairment is **organic** or **functional**, or **permanent** or **transient** (**Diplock**).

Cap 224 of the Penal Code (Singapore)
Section 84
Nothing is an offence which is done by a person who at the time of doing it by reason of unsoundness of mind is incapable of knowing the nature of the act or that he is doing what is either wrong or contrary to law.

Section 85(2)
Intoxication shall be a defence to any criminal charges if by reason thereof the person charged at the time of the act or omission complained of did not know that such act or omission was wrong or did not know what he was doing and

(a) the state of intoxication was caused without his consent by malicious or negligent act or another person, or
(b) the person charged was by reason of intoxication insane temporarily or otherwise at the time of such act or omission.

In Singapore, Section 84 has been treated as being the same as the McNaughton Rules. "**Unsoundness of mind**" is not defined and has been employed on the one hand to mean the **medical concept of psychosis** and on the other hand to mean the **legal concept of insanity**. A psychotic in the medical sense need not be insane in the legal sense. Similarly, a person who is legally insane need not be medically psychotic because unsoundness of mind in local practice has been extended to cover persons who are defective in reason from mental retardation. Confusion arises when medical psychosis is equated with legal insanity.

Diminished Responsibility

The defence of diminished responsibility is available only if the charge is murder. It is often pleaded because murder is punishable with death and a successful plea under exception 7 to Section 300 of the Penal Code will reduce the sentence to a definite term of imprisonment.

Exception 7 to Section 300 of the Penal Code

"Culpable homicide is not murder if the offender was suffering from such **abnormality of mind** (whether arising from a condition of arrested or retarded development of mind or any inherent causes or induced by disease or injury) as **substantially impaired** his **mental responsibility** for his acts and omissions in causing the death or being a party to causing the death."

The psychiatrist is involved in establishing the cause of "abnormality of mind".

Lord Parker C. J. defines "**abnormality of mind**" as "[...] a state of mind so different from that of ordinary human beings that the **reasonable man** [...] would term it abnormal. It appears to us wide enough to cover the mind's activities in all its aspects, not only the perception of physical acts and matters, and the ability to form a rational judgement as to whether the act was right or wrong, but also the ability to exercise will-power to control physical acts in accordance with that rational judgement."

It is important to note that abnormality is a **lay concept** and the "mind" includes **impulse control** as well.

Misuse of Drugs Act (Cap 185, 2008 Rev Ed) — MDA

In Singapore, drug-related offences can lead to the imposition of the death penalty. However, there are three categories of drug-related offenders who may escape capital punishment.

1. If the accused can prove that he/she is nothing more than a "courier", on the balance of probabilities and according to strict definitions and criteria, he/she may not be sentenced to death. (However, there is no mention of knowledge and intention involved.)
2. If the public prosecutor certifies that the accused has "substantively assisted" the Central Narcotic Bureau in disrupting drug trafficking activities within or outside Singapore (i.e., substantive assistance limb), he/she would qualify for discretionary diminished responsibility but not exempted from punishment.
3. The diminished responsibility limb can be extended to the accused when justified by psychiatric examination and opinion.

B. Criminal Procedure Code

Remand for psychiatric assessment*   (Pre-trial)
Fitness to plead or stand trial   (At trial)
Detention under Minister's Order   (Unfit for trial or
Review or discharge by Visitors Board   Post trial detention)

*In bailable offence, the accused may not be remanded but should be produced in court when fit to stand trial.

The **Visitors Board** must review those who are detained due to unsoundness of mind at least once in six months to determine their mental state and make suitable recommendations regarding fitness to plead, discharge, or further detention.

Criteria on Fitness to Plead

Capability of:

a. understanding what is the charge
b. knowing the difference between pleading guilty and not guilty
c. following the court proceedings
d. challenging the jurors (jury system abolished in Singapore)
e. instructing legal counsels

In reality, fitness to plead is fairly relative.

MENTAL DISORDERS AND TREATMENT ACT (MDTA) Revised 1985

The MDTA is split up and repealed by:

Mental Health (Care and Treatment) Act 2008

Mental Capacity Act 2008

Mandatory Treatment Order (2010, CPC)

Mental Health (Care and Treatment) Act 2008 (MHCTA)

The Act consists of 3 parts:

Part I
Preliminary

Sections 1 and 2

Part II
Admission and Detention of Mentally Disordered Persons in Psychiatric Institution

Sections 3 to 22

Part III
General Provisions

Sections 23 to 34

Mental Capacity Act 2008 (MCA)

Explanatory Statement:

This Act seeks to reform and update the law where decisions need to be made on behalf of **adults lacking capacity**. The Act will govern **decision-making** on behalf of adults, both where they lose mental capacity at some point in their lives (e.g., as a result of dementia or brain injury) and where the incapacitating condition has been present since birth. It covers a wide range of decisions, on **personal welfare** and **financial matters** and **substitute decision-making** by **attorneys** or **court-appointed "deputies"**, and clarifies the position where no such formal process has been adopted. The Act provides **recourse**, where **necessary**, to a court with power to deal with personal welfare and financial decisions on behalf of adults lacking capacity.

It is administered by the Office of Public Guardian and the Mental Capacity Court.

This Act consists of 9 parts:

Part I
Preliminary

Sections 1 and 2

Part II
Persons Who Lack Capacity

Sections 3 to 6

Part III
Acts in Connection with Care and Treatment

Sections 7 to 10

Part IV
Lasting Powers of Attorney

Sections 11 to 18

Part V
General Powers of Court and Appointment of Deputies

Sections 19 to 25

Part VI
Excluded Decisions and Declaratory Provisions

Sections 26 to 29

Part VII
Public Guardian and Board of Visitors

Sections 30 to 34

Part VIII
Supplementary Powers, Practice, and Procedure of Court

Sections 35 to 39

Part IX
Miscellaneous

Sections 40 to 42

In the **MHCTA** and **MCA**, there is no mention of "unsoundness of mind". Instead, "mentally disordered person" with attendant conditions or criteria is used.

Under **MCA Part 2: Persons Who Lack Capacity**, the key principles which apply to **decisions** and **actions** taken under the Act are that a person must be **assumed** to have capacity until it is proved otherwise. He must also be **supported** to make his own decisions as far as it is practicable to do so. He is not to be treated as lacking capacity to make decisions simply because he has made **unwise** decisions before. In other words, he has the **right** to make **irrational** or **eccentric** decisions that others may judge to not be in his best interest. However, everything done or every decision made under that Act for a person who lacks capacity must be done **in his best interest**.

The definition for a person who lacks capacity for the purposes of the Act focuses on the **particular time** when a decision has to be made and on a **particular matter** to which **the decision relates**, rather than on any theoretical ability to make decisions generally. It follows that a person can lack capacity for the purposes of the Act even if the **loss of capacity** is **partial** or **temporary** or if his capacity **fluctuates**. It also follows that a person may lack capacity in relation to one matter but not in relation to another matter.

The inability to make a decision must be caused by an **impairment of** or **disturbance in** the **functioning of the mind or brain**. This could cover a range of problems, such as **psychiatric illness**, **learning disability**, **dementia**, or **brain damage**, that affect the functioning of the mind or brain and cause the person to be unable to make the decision. When lack of capacity has been determined, then the **relevant part(s)** of MCA that follow may be implemented.

The person involved is usually aged **21 or over**. He would be deemed unable to make a decision if he is deficient in any one of the following abilities:

1. Must be able to comprehend the information relevant to the decision
2. Must be able to retain this information
3. Must be able to weigh and use it to arrive at a choice
4. Must be able to communicate the decision in any way

In ascertaining a person's best interest, all relevant circumstances and factors must be considered and balanced in order to determine what would be in the best interest of the person concerned.

In **Part IV** of the **MCA**, a new statutory form of power of attorney is created viz. the "**lasting power of attorney**" (**LPA**). By making an LPA, an individual (the **donor**) confers on another individual (**donee**) authority to make decisions about the **donor's personal welfare**, **property** and **affairs**, or **specified matters** concerning those areas when the donor no longer has capacity to make such decisions. The donor must be aged 18 or over and have the capacity to execute an LPA. Rules regulating making an LPA for donors and donees must be complied with.

Mandatory Treatment Order 2010 (MTO) [CPC — Sections 338–339]

The abnormal offender is judged according to whether he is legally of sound or unsound mind, which has led to outcomes of limited disposal. Over the years, there has been a loosening of this rigid approach with a better understanding of offenders and their offences, resulting in more therapeutic sentencings. The MTO is one of several community-based sentences **in lieu of imprisonment**. Offenders who are mentally ill may be remanded up to 3 weeks for assessment by an **appointed psychiatrist** at IMH. Suitability with inclusion and exclusion criteria is determined and forwarded to the court for decision to mandate. Treatment periods of up to 2 years with regular follow-ups and court reportings must be observed and administered by IMH.

In general, receiving a MTO would imply that the offence is not of a serious nature and related to a mental condition that is not severe and is **treatable**. **Personality disorders**, **addictive behaviours**, **mental retardation**, and **severe impulsive** and **mental disorders** are **excluded**. Offenders must be agreeable to accept and pay for the treatment. On completion of treatment or when in default, the matter is referred back to the court for further action.

Consent

Consent is required from the patient in a number of situations, such as when requesting for a medical report when confidentiality is breached or for invasive investigation and treatment procedures.

Fitness to give consent depends on the minimal age of the individual as set by the law, the mental state of the patient, the level of understanding that the individual is capable of, and the necessity of the life-saving measure. In the UK, no one but the individual can give consent. However, in Singapore, the next of kin or guardians can give consent in good faith on behalf of their wards when necessary. When in doubt, the advice of the Attorney General should be sought.

Assessment for Litigation/Compensation

A quick and simple approach is to ask the following questions:

1. What is the nature of the lesion, injury, or disorder caused?
2. What is the consequence of the lesion, injury, or disorder?
3. What is the reaction to the lesion, injury, or disorder?

4. What is the reaction to the consequence of the lesion, injury, or disorder?
5. What is the contribution of the personality to the reactions?
6. What is the consequent influence on the personality?
7. What are the advantages or benefits derived from the symptom or disability?

Punitive or Therapeutic in Approach

In the past, sentencing of convicted offenders is restricted to the issue of whether they are of sound or unsound mind. The disposal is limited. However, there has been a better appreciation of the grey area in terms of the responsibility of those who are intellectually challenged or mentally ill. The approach now is more humane and therapeutic.

Generally speaking, depending on the stage of development, value system, and availability of resources, society may **medicalise** some deviant or antisocial behaviours and treat them or **criminalise** such behaviours and punish the individuals responsible. Thus, drug problems may come under the Ministry of Home Affairs or the Ministry of Health in different countries.

Charts

- Mental Health (Care and Treatment) Act 2008
- Criminal Procedure Code 2010

Guide to Forensic Examination (and Medical Report)

- Sound clinical foundations and objective investigation skills are fundamental.
- All persons giving evidence are officers of court helping to seek the truth.

Mental Health (Care and Treatment) Act 2008

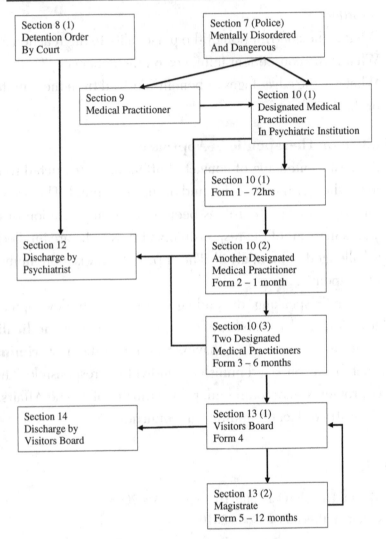

- All responses are directed to the Court (i.e., the presiding Magistrate/ Judge).
- The Forensic Psychiatrist is neither for the Prosecution nor for the Defence.
- The Expert Witness-Accused relationship replaces the Doctor-Patient relationship.

Criminal Procedure Code 2010

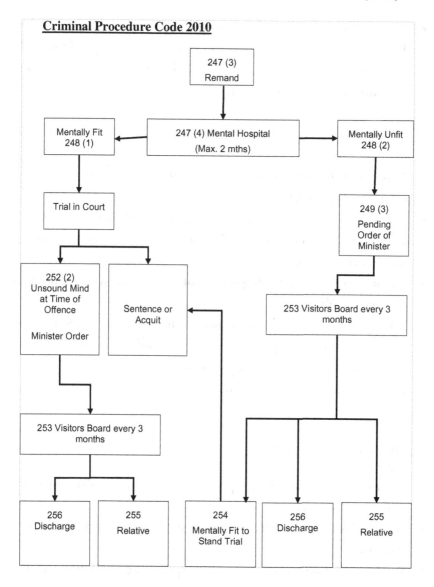

- Information or evidence obtained can be used against the Accused.
- Remember the "first oath" of "do no harm."
- Always ask "what are the **facts of the case**" and do not rely on hearsay or interpretation.
- History taking/clerking from reliable informants and sources should be systematic, thorough, detailed, and chronological (and to include drugs and alcohol).

- **Be specific** in the date, day, time, place, person, and any other data.
- The more detailed, chronological, consistent in repeat history the more likely **factual** In the process **consistency**, **memory** and **mental state** at material point of time assessed could/would exclude organic conditions.
- **Inconsistency** in accounts during repeated interviews may indicate **malingering**.
- Determine the **presence of mental disorder**, in particular **psychosis** and **intellectual disability**
- Is it present **before, during**, or **after** the legal issues concerned?
- Presence of psychosis or intellectual disability is essential for unsoundness of mind.
- Unsoundness of mind is **legal insanity** and is not synonymous with **clinical psychosis**.
- A psychotic need not be of unsound mind and severe intellectual disability (though not psychotic) can be considered to be of unsound mind according to the legal criteria involved.
- **Dementia** would be of unsound mind when acting under psychotic symptoms.

Opinions:

- **First offenders** have better prognosis than **repeat offenders** with different offences.
- Balance "**untruthful till proven otherwise**" against "**benefit of doubt**".
- Evidence and opinion on criminal responsibility is **at the point of time** of **commission**.
- Sometimes **unsoundness of mind** is considered when the psychotic denies wrongdoing but justifies actions based on hallucinations and/ or delusions.
- Fitness to plead or stand trial is **at the point of time** of **assessment**.

- Soundness or unsoundness of mind is virtually defined by **legal criteria**.
- Explanation (or a causal link) does not equate to exoneration/exculpation.

WRITING MEDICAL REPORTS

- The content and comprehensiveness of a report is variable depending on prevalent practice and expectations or requirements.
- Medical reports should be concise, precise, and therefore not lengthy (the longer the report, the more mistakes there likely would be).
- It is akin to the abstract of a complete article.
- One learns to focus on what is important and relevant.
- One learns to be clear, organised, and specific.
- One learns to use correct and appropriate words or expressions.
- Avoid subjective adverbs and adjectives; every word must be defensible.
- Recommendations and mitigation should be suggested when appropriate.

8 Active Balance and Passive Equilibrium

It seems that there are **three major areas** of **conflict**, **tension**, and **stress** in modern living. They are not mutually exclusive and in fact overlap and interplay. What is discussed below is with special reference to psychotherapy. Indeed, these conflicts or dilemmas are applicable to other things.

A. Evolutionary Processes versus Revolutionary Changes

Biological development is evolutionary in nature and its functioning is integrative. There is a built-in feedback mechanism that monitors the organism's internal and external environments continuously. Biological processes generally follow a predictable course and timespan. Thus, the growth and development of a child go through defined stages. Education and training take time and specialisation even more. There is no way to mass produce precious personnel in a shorter time by way of mechanisation, computerisation, and automation, which are the key processes in productivity. Hence, foreign talents are imported when needs arise. Soon, however, habit and inbreeding take place and become a problem. The local workforce may or may not be ready but is picky, impatient, and feels displaced and resentful.

Social changes on the other hand are man-made and tend to be ad hoc and lopsided, directing at specific problems and needs during certain periods of time. In our competitive world, they occur so rapidly that our biological make-up cannot match the pace. A concrete example would be the phenomenon of jet-lag when our physiological rhythm is out of step with changes in time zone. The necessity for shift duties, especially the third shift, apart from social implications, can also upset bodily systems with regard to sleep, appetite, and bowel habits. It is not surprising that sleeping pills and alcohol are used to overcome the problem of insomnia. Frequent abrupt changes of policy and organisation disrupt people in their long-term plans and commitments. This is made worse by incredible advances in technology. Old jobs are destroyed and new jobs are created. Soon, foreign talents or workers would be replaced by computers, machines, and robots.

Biological adaptation takes time and learning processes are arduous. They cannot be reversed or switched on and off at will. The older generation or elderly persons in particular suffer because they have greater difficulty coping with rapid changes, acquiring new know-how, or undergoing upgrading or re-training. Even conversion to the metric system was a laborious process and took years to complete. Cultural attitudes, beliefs, and customs are not changed overnight by economic success or scientific discovery. The human mind may reach into the sky to be among gods, but the human heart is still in the jungle with the animals.

Implications for Psychotherapy

Modern living is fast-paced and changing, characterised by the culture of instant gratification, constant stimulation, seduction, and self-indulgence with fads and fashion, the internet, sex, drugs, and virtual reality. However, psychotherapy takes time and the individual needs time, but changes do not keep time.

On the other hand, deep-rooted cultural beliefs and practices are not to be underestimated for their therapeutic roles. They can be an alliance or an enemy in therapy.

B. Role Prescription/Acceptance versus Individual Right/ Freedom

In Confucian society, there is an **ethical code of conduct** and a **hierarchy of social organisation** that must be strictly observed. Everybody knows his station in life and lives according to his **multiple roles** — as a ruler, citizen, employer, employee, friend, father, son, brother, husband, and so on. When he acts dutifully and in line with expectations, there is order. Naturally, this is subject to complete and willing acceptance of prescribed roles inculcated from young. The elders must always be respected and their words are law. Young men and women who have come of age must marry and the go-between is asked to look for compatible matches. The greatest sin of lack of filial piety is to not produce a male heir to carry on the family name. For the female, she must follow her father before she is married, follow her husband when she is married, and follow her son when she is widowed. She must also be virtuous in her conduct, appearance, speech, and work. There seems no place for self-identity and expression. It is to be expected that there will be sufferings and tragedies mostly because of **human weakness** and **wickedness**, rather than the system itself, **as roles are abused and exploited for selfish ends by those in positions of power**.

But with exposure to western philosophy and way of life, men and women apparently liberate themselves from social restrictions and claim their **rights as individuals** to seek self-fulfilment or do as they please. The gender or seniority of a person do not seem to matter much. In western society, people call one another by personal name regardless of differences in hierarchy and generation. This reduces all relationships to a linear one of apparent equality and contributes to social chaos. Conflict arises when people's **expression of freedom** is at odds with their **social obligations**. It becomes disastrous when they cannot handle their freedom responsibly and abuse it; then it is like the autonomous cancer cell that grows and multiplies indiscriminately until the host body is destroyed. Inevitably, respect for law and order and traditional wisdom breaks down. Schism and alienation set in. Seniority and experience count for nothing. The filial children of yesterday become unwanted parents of today. The new idolatry is indiscriminate **individualism**.

Of course, man would like to believe that he is enlightened through education and religion. However, cruelty, corruption, and crime still abound everywhere. Only the form and method have become more sophisticated. Countries are divided among themselves by ideology, race, language, and religion. They kill each other in the loftiest proclamation. The violence of exploding bombs, greed in drug trafficking, and exploitation of sex regardless of consequences and conscience complete the scenario. Human nature over the ages has been unchanging. However, to shackle a person into rigid roles is as dangerous and tragic as to give free rein to his passions.

Implications for Psychotherapy

Whether we admit it or not, we play **multiple roles** and interact at **many levels** consciously or unconsciously all the time. At different times and in different situations, there may be a dominant role and other subsidiary roles. The doctor and patient roles in a clinical setting are dominant roles. When other roles creep in between them, transference is said to take place and the relationship is changed.

It is often forgotten that the **relationship** between two persons changes with change in roles. Furthermore, the characteristics or expectations of each role also undergo changes. Each society has its own concept of the necessity and expectation of roles. However, in real life, certain hierarchical roles are unalterable. People do not just relate and interact as equal individuals but also observe their social stations. There is genuine **conflict** between preserving family structure and functioning and establishing individual identity and independence.

C. Survival of the Misfits and Unfits (and Unwilling)

It should be stated from the outset that the right to survival is unquestionable. The terms "misfits" and "unfits" are not absolute and have nothing to do with the Nazi concept of creating a superior race. They are to be viewed from the perspective of the biological concept of Darwinism regarding the **survival of the fittest**. In some sense, we are all misfits, unfit, and unwilling to some extent. Our personality development is **uneven** and we all have our strengths and weaknesses. We may be brilliant or dull in mind, beautiful or blemished in physique, or stable or volatile in temperament. An individual could be an intellectual giant but suffer from social inadequacies, sexual deviance, or emotional immaturity. To put it crudely, there are people who are socially high class but morally low class, intellectually first class but spiritually no class. Depending on the period and culture he lives in and the value system that is upheld, he may enjoy public prominence or languish in anonymity. **One man's meat may be another man's poison, but what is meat today may be poison tomorrow.**

To achieve progress, we have traded **general versatility** for **intensive specialisation**. In the process, we have become increasingly **interdependent** for mutual services but also increasingly vulnerable when such services break down or when our individual talents fail or go out of demand. On the other hand, **market forces** are such that what is in demand can dictate exorbitant terms with impunity. There are very young millionaires or even billionaires with their innovations or creations that capture the world.

With advancements in medical sciences and technology as well as the affluence of civilised society, the **frail** and **feeble** in **body**, **mind**, and **morals** are more capable of surviving. They not only survive without being productive but also expect better quality of life and services encouraged by the welfare state. People with personality disorders or mental and behavioural disorders, abusers of psychoactive substances, the physically and intellectually disabled or handicapped, and the aged or sick would all fall under this category. They are not only a stress to themselves as consumers, but also a stress to others as providers. Incidentally, it is ironic that while fortunes are spent on modern medicine to prolong some dying lives, fortunes are also made from arms sales to exterminate lives. When man plays god, he must deal with the devil. Ageing populations with declining birthrates are going to be a monstrous problem. Less and less people who are productive will have to support more and more people who are unproductive.

Implications for Psychotherapy

Psychotherapy would have to grapple with issues of values, judgement, morality, economics, and politics. In developed countries, the pressure is on the welfare state, but for other less developed countries, the burden is on the family.

What are the Answers?

Human solutions to problems are always at the expense of something else; every solution creates a new problem. There is no perfect or permanent solution as **a price must be paid by someone, somewhere, sometime**. Nevertheless, suffering must be alleviated.

In terms of psychodynamics and treatment, western psycho-therapy aims at not only removing symptoms but also promoting growth and development of the individual. It is patient-centred and the interests of others are of secondary importance. This is consistent with the belief that individual rights are sacrosanct. Eastern society is family-centred and the individual is expected to put the interests of the group above those of the self. For ages, the Chinese have also coped by accepting their individual fate and destiny when faced with trials and tribulations, which allows individual failure or weakness to be overlooked and makes life more bearable.

It may be said that western society encourages vertical development of individuals which then spurs horizontal growth of the community. But the eastern philosophy of life emphasises the wellbeing of the whole through the selfless contributions of individuals. There is a Chinese saying that when there is no country or nation, there is no family or home. Perhaps the answer lies in the:

ACTIVE BALANCE (win-win) of OPPOSITE VIRTUES
and **NOT** the
PASSIVE EQUILIBRIUM (zero sum) of DOMINATION and
RESIGNATION.

The human community is made up of individuals and the individuals cannot be effective without the community. Perhaps we need a culture that can **restrain the "Id", relax the "Super-ego"**, and **reinforce the "Ego"**, which would then hold all things together in harmony. Psychotherapy must therefore recognise the cultural norms, values, and realities from which the patient comes and to which the patient returns.

9 Stress, Mental Health, and Management

As everything in life is relevant to mental health and psychiatry, mental health and psychiatry are relevant to everyone.

Stress is part of life. In this competitive world, however, some say that it is or should be a way of life. Stress is therefore unavoidable, but it is **not always necessary**. Very often, it is the result of incompetent, mediocre, selfish, and greedy management or personality problems. A hidden or higher reason for stress to be created is perhaps to toughen people up to ensure survival, but then there will be casualties even before going to war. There are both **intrinsic** and **extrinsic factors** involved in stress. The **nature of mental health work** requires that the psychiatrist should be well **informed** and **interested** about **life**.

The Coil Spring and the Load

Individuals are like coil springs of different material, thickness, length, and strength. Each time a weight is suspended, the spring stretches and as the load is increased, the spring will stretch proportionally. When the weight is removed, the spring returns to its original state. However, if the load keeps increasing, the spring will keep stretching. There comes a point where the spring does not quite return to its original position when the weight is taken off. This can also happen when a certain weight is applied over a prolonged or indefinite period of time. In this instance, the spring has undergone a qualitative change and lost its full resilience. Subsequently, its response to the force applied would be erratic and difficult to predict. Eventually, with increasing load, a critical point is reached when the spring snaps, like the final straw that breaks the camel's back.

Of course, an excessive weight right from the start or at any point thereafter would produce the same result in a more dramatic fashion. However, if the whole process is carried out in a different medium, such as when it is immersed in a liquid, then the buoyancy effect will affect the response of the spring to the applied force.

The Horse, the Cart, and the Road

Putting "the cart before the horse" refers to the wrong sequence of doing things or adopting the wrong priorities. Here, we are concerned about productivity.

Carrying a certain load from A to B within a certain time frame will depend on the nature of the load, the power of the horse, the size of the cart, and the conditions of the road. There are several variables that are relevant to this task, but we will not discuss them all.

When the horsepower is fixed, there will be a maximal limit to payload. The horse pulls easily when the cart is small and the load is light. More often than not, it is a full load, but within limits the horse can still do a good job even though its reserves may be reached. Crisis comes when the cart is overloaded or expanded to carry more and no additional horse is available. This calls for a decision as to what valuable load should be carried and what dispensable load should be discarded, but this is not always done.

Sometimes, the horse matches the cart and the load, but the road can be narrow, winding, and uneven. When a time schedule needs to be strictly followed, the horse and the cart will end up breaking down from exhaustion and making extra trips. In modern IT language, we know that every computer has a fixed capacity and speed. When the hard disk is full, it cannot take in more data. But the human workforce seems to have no limits to capacity and speed to meet production targets.

The Driver and The Car

The performance of the car on the road depends not only on its road-worthiness and the traffic conditions but also on the way it is driven. There are drivers who drive without changing gears, with the foot on the clutch, or with the hand brake on. One can imagine the serious wear and tear, wastage of energy with much heat and exhaust, and eventual breakdown of the engine and parts. The new autopilot electric car will lead to atrophy of driving skills.

Sloggers and Shirkers

With emphasis on paper qualifications and performance measured in selective quantifiable units, the phenomenon of apparent quality and quantity emerges. Qualifications do not always predict delivery as there are other important factors at play, such as personality, character, commitment, health status, and energy level. However, meritocracy often develops into elitism and mistakes made during recruitment might be concealed.

Thus, on paper, the staff complement may be full and everyone receives the same reward, but in reality, there may be only 7–8 out of 10 who pull their weight and 2–3 who are not doing their part. To achieve the productivity of 10 employees, the 7–8 "sloggers" would have to put in extra to make up for the 2–3 "shirkers". The management, which is concerned with increasing its output, therefore depends more and more on the sloggers for their input. While the shirkers are allowed to get away, the sloggers are under stress as they have to do well above their share and wind up feeling resentful. The sloggers also suffer when rules are tightened with the shirkers in mind.

Stress is further aggravated when the management, to put it crudely, is preoccupied with "projecting an image" and "covering its backside", which generate unproductive activities and waste resources. The worldly wise soon recognises that the priority is not so much to provide a better service but to please those in authority. Amazingly, feedback, monitoring, auditing, and accountability appear to be satisfied merely by making rhetoric statements and submitting questionable figures. The paradoxical outcome is that the more capable the individual, the more is expected from him, the more he is under stress, and the more likely he will break down when he remains in the system, even when suitably rewarded. Stress becomes poisonous when the slogger works under a shirker whose output depends on the former's input.

Input and Output

It is not often appreciated that the output of the management depends on the input from the ground. As such, when the individual's input goes to his own output and does not directly contribute to the management's output or image, then his performance is not likely to be recognised and rewarded. Increased mechanisation, automation, and computerisation are intended to increase production, but productivity depends on trained people.

In this age of information technology, computerisation is an answer to efficiency and productivity. Facts and figures, when required by the management, are displayed immediately at the touch of the finger, but it requires a sufficient number of people at the bottom to regularly collate and key in the necessary data. Computerisation does not reduce the workforce. The user depends on the feeder, and although people at the top may take minutes to formulate and issue ideas or instructions, it still takes others hours, days, or weeks to process and accomplish. Often the results are obvious, redundant, or inconsequential and much time, effort, and money are wasted at the expense of other priorities. However, the management must be seen as working and protocol must be observed.

Apart from production targets and deadlines, people may also find themselves trapped to do things against their convictions and principles. To opt out would mean unemployment and privation.

Self Interest and Group Interest

Self interest is innate and natural and has survival value. The group is composed of individuals and group interest should be to enhance individual interest and survival. However, there are many kinds of groups and each group has its own purpose or function, characteristics, and life. As each individual can be a member of more than one group, there will be conflicts of interest and loyalty. People have their own priority of membership and hierarchy of group interest. Generally speaking, that which provides work and livelihood is usually the most important.

When basic needs are satisfied, people look beyond towards higher living standards, better working conditions, career development, job satisfaction, and being somebody. Once again, there will be conflicts and tension. Stress is aggravated when group interest is divided, undermined by self interest, or controlled by interests outside the group. It should be noted that there are often subgroups with their own specific interests within the larger group. Sometimes, the purpose and function of the group may become outdated and its continuity becomes a sentimental burden.

History of Corporate Stress

Corporate stress existed since ancient times. There have been strong but bad rulers as well as good but weak ones. There have been ambitious and scheming courtiers who manipulated emperors and exploited the people, and there have also been capable and virtuous statesmen who were banished or executed. From a historical perspective, an enlightened dictator who is superego-guided may be better than a mediocre democracy that is id-driven.

In modern management and governance, the top priority is to be in control via whatever means and methods (powered perhaps by branded MBAs — mind brain altered or automated). It has been said that management creates jobs for itself and work for others. Indeed, the management size often grows faster than the core business manpower. The management does not contribute directly to productivity but devises ways and measurements to squeeze their work horses to produce more. The management seems to engage in regular travelling to get ideas, lengthy meetings to promote ideas, top-down delegation to enforce ideas, and remote controlling instead of walking the talk. What is achieved is usually "image creation" and "backside covering". It is not unlike a parasite that takes control of the host and drains off much of the harvest of labour to feed its separate existence, infrastructure, and running costs. The work horses are further squeezed to provide for the CEO's bonuses and the stakeholders' benefits. Talent and quality or standards are dispensable if they do not meet the prevailing culture and expectations of the management. Therefore, it is the consolidation of power and control that really matters for the management. For others who have acquired invaluable experience and wisdom over the course of work, they are soon discarded at a cutoff point because they are considered obstacles to the compulsive need for change and the need to make way for rejuvenation. The cycle of three steps forward and two steps back in terms of experience and wisdom are repeated and seen as progress as long as power and control are maintained.

Thinking within the Box

Thinking within the box is natural when it is downloaded like software onto a hard disk and one is constrained to think only in terms of its contents. When the content is "I know all, I know best, I decide all, I veto the rest", the consequence is "fear to speak, foolish to speak, futile to speak". ISOs, SOPs, and NUTS (the "No U-Turn Syndrome") are orders of the day. To think out of the box, we need more boxes with different contents mixing freely. However, too many shortsighted free ideas and demands may have dire long-term consequences.

Prohibition and Permissiveness

In conservative or prohibitive culture and society, values, attitudes, beliefs, and customs are clearly spelled out. There is little ambiguity on what is good or bad and what is right or wrong. Rules are established to prevent the undesirable from taking place and people are therefore more inhibited. In liberal or permissive cultures and societies, boundaries of good versus bad and right versus wrong are blurred; rules are not absolute and people are more adventurous and experimenting.

However, prohibition does not prevent what is undesirable from happening, and when bad things do happen, solutions are often limited and restrictive. Where there is permissiveness, things are allowed to happen, but solutions are more quickly found to deal with the various problems that surface. For instance, sex is associated with procreation and the transmission of sexually transmitted diseases (STDs). The surest way to avoid unnecessary procreation and STDs is to prohibit sex. That is, when there are no unwanted pregnancies or STDs, there is no reason to have interventions. However, when promiscuity is a way of life, one can indulge in sex without getting into trouble so to speak by learning about the safe periods, contraception, and the treatments available. Thus, open society seems more innovative, creative, and advanced. When closed society is faced with problems, it has to look to the open society for solutions.

Innovation needs to be encouraged with support and flexibility, but it should also be tempered with conscience and caution to prevent harms.

The Economic Preoccupation

In the modern world, the new dictator that drives us on and on is materialism or consumerism. Making money has become an important part of our culture because of its purchasing power. It can even buy talents and citizenship. There are so many things that are attractive, desirable, and irresistible. Furthermore, these things are churned out so fast that they are being replaced continuously. To delay in getting them means missing out on them for good. The pace is such that he who postpones or procrastinates in his gratification is a loser. The race is on and everyone takes the shortest and quickest routes to achieve their objectives by hook or by crook. Not surprisingly, advanced credit, competition, conflict, conspiracy, confrontation, and even criminal behaviour have occurred. Short-term interests prevail. Instead of being a byproduct of what one can afford, lifestyles become the end-product to have at all cost. As a result, economic pursuit supersedes human values and relationships. There is no more altruism or higher calling.

The Customer is Always Right

The emphasis that the customer is always right is both misleading and a source of stress and mental health problems to those who serve in the front line. What it really means is that the customer has money and we want him or her to spend on our goods and services now or in the future. So, if he or she does not buy today, it is hoped that he or she will buy tomorrow and will keep coming back to do so. Thus, the statement should honestly be that money is always right provided it is not illegally derived. To insist that the customer is always right is to say that there are no personality dysfunctions or difficulties as understood in psychiatry or persons with negative social traits.

There is another context where the clients or consumers, particularly the users of government services, are also always right. In this case, it is not directly related to economic performance. The causes and costs of complaints may affect political outcomes, such as voting. Thus, complaints, whether they are reasonable or unreasonable, are feared by both honest and corrupt governments.

The Amoeba and the Specialised Cell

Although the amoeba is a lowly unicellular organism, it is free and independent. It moves, seeks food, grows, and reproduces itself. Life for the amoeba goes on in monotonous cycles. Only multicellular organisms are capable of higher quality of life.

The more complex the differentiation and organisation of cells into tissues, organs, and systems, the more developed and versatile the organism. However, the individual cell has to sacrifice its independence and mobility to serve a specific function. The specialised cell then serves a greater purpose for the benefit of the whole organism.

However, every now and then, some cells decide to go their own way regardless of the consequences. They proliferate autonomously, spread from organ to organ, and are in fact cancerous. Eventually, they harm or kill the host body and themselves (it is therefore important to detect cancer early and treat it radically). Man in society has the dilemma of preserving his individuality and independence, like the amoeba, or fulfilling prescribed social roles, like the specialised cell. Stress arises when the two interests are in conflict.

The Soloist and the Orchestra

The aim of many musicians is to be able to perform as soloists. However, the music made by a soloist cannot compare with that of an orchestra in terms of grandeur, richness, and impact. To make great symphonic music, every player from the first violin to the percussionist must play their part accordingly and follow the directions of the conductor. Every instrument, every note, and every pause has a specific place. There is no such thing as outplaying one another in loudness or in speed or reaching a compromise. Competition does exist, but only to determine the best players who can lead each section to bring the performance to the highest plane possible. In concertos, the star player is the soloist and he is accompanied by the whole orchestra. The conductor controls the orchestral players to coordinate with the soloist. They will play as one to create the desired music.

The music that each orchestra is capable of performing depends on its size and component players. To perform well, the orchestra needs time to practise and rehearse. Frequent changes to programmes, musical scores, or conductors will affect its performance. To have good music, we also need the necessary support, environment, and atmosphere.

Inclusiveness and Exclusiveness

People are always more important than systems because the human element is always crucial. Life is a relationship between cells that form tissues; between tissues that form organs; between organs that form systems; and between systems that form the complete organism.

The highest form of relationship is non-self-seeking love, or love that is inclusive and grows and makes the whole. It is not technical, intellectual, or professional, and it enlarges its circle of relationships between persons, families, neighbourhoods, communities, and nations. Opposing it is exclusiveness, or the drive to set ourselves apart from others perhaps for efficiency or excellence. Being distinct, it discriminates, divides, dominates, and demoralises. The in-group, however, fosters identity, comradeship, and loyalty. If it could be more inclusive rather than exclusive, then its growth and strength would know no boundaries. **The secret of successful management lies in the in-group that is inclusive**. Through sharing and belonging, it inspires solidarity and puts the common or greater good first.

Vision and Mission

It is fashionable if not mandatory for every institution or organisation to have a vision and mission statement. Hence, many heads will meet for hours and days to craft and recraft these statements, which become the ends themselves and exist mostly on paper. Implementation is either neglected or compromised. It is not unlike the section leader of each instrument coming together to compose a perfect symphony that is beyond the capabilities of the orchestra while the audience is starving for some music to be played.

Policy and Traffic Lights

Policy is like traffic lights. When green, traffic flows smoothly, but when it suddenly turns red, accidents and casualties happen. Then when it changes to green again, the traffic in front will begin to move while those behind will follow slowly. After the last general elections (2011), a "new normal" came about. People at the top quickly responded more openly and inclusively, but the middle rung reacted tardily and the lower end hardly moved. If the lights change erratically, there will be traffic jams and chaos.

Helicopter View and Submarine View

Much emphasis has been given to the importance of possessing a helicopter view. The helicopter view sees far and wide and what is on the surface, but to see what is below the surface, a submarine view is needed. As the saying goes, people who live in ivory towers are out of touch with the reality on the ground, or they merely act as messengers of misinformation.

The Means and The Ends

It has been said by Soren Kierkegaard that "the end does not justify the means for the means is an end itself", presumably even if the end is something good.

Human solutions to problems are always at the expense of something else. Every solution creates new problems as a price must be paid by someone, somewhere, sometime. When we cure disease and promote health, we increase lifespans and face ageing populations. When we develop the economy and create wealth, we also generate waste and pollution. As the name of the game is "progress and prosperity", we must create wealth in order to develop, and to create more wealth, we must compete for consumers, which leads to environmental destruction and more waste. Our standard of living is measured by the amount of junk mail in the letter box and reusable material in the garbage bin.

There are two sides to every virtue or vice depending on the circumstance and perspective. That is, what is virtue in one context may be vice in another and vice versa. It is important to observe rules and regulations, but sometimes it is more important to bend them (although rules should be rules and exceptions remain exceptions). A staff member who works overtime may be diligent, but he or she may also inconvenience others and incur higher costs. Perfectionism can be an asset or a setback. As the saying goes, what is meat to one may be poison to another. Furthermore, what is meat today may be poison tomorrow and vice versa. There is also a Chinese saying that the wheel of fortune turns round and round, and thus there is hope of change in life.

The Square One Theory

There is a saying that too many cooks spoil the broth.
To solve the "problem", a team consisting of a head chef, assistant cooks, and kitchen hands is formed.
Thereafter, the team meets regularly to discuss the menu and recipe.

Members are also sent for courses and training.

With high expectations, more and more new menus and recipes are created.

Eventually, a glossy cookbook is produced and accepted.

However, the broth is still not served because the cooks are not cooking and there are no ingredients in the pantry.

Evolution of Knowledge

When we are young, we see only grey

As we grow and learn, we distinguish between black and white

Upon becoming adults, we realise the shades of grey in between

Then there are experts who can detect black in white and white in black

There are also others who argue that black is white and white is black

Of course, there will be a few who decide what is black and what is white

In the end, it is all grey again

There are no limits to human intelligence and rationalisation.

Schizophrenic Statistics and Knowledge

As knowledge increases and what was untreatable in the past becomes treatable, there is also the trend of changing thresholds in criteria and definitions of disease. As a result, a high percentage of the population would be suffering from every disease or disorder ever known. If one were to add up all the percentages or rates of each physical disease or mental disorder published, then everyone would have had to suffer from more than one illness. There would be no healthy individuals and everyone would end up taking medicines and health supplements.

On the other hand, there are 24 hours in the day. Physiologically, the body needs regular meals, exercise, recreation, and 6–8 hours of sleep on average to stay healthy and function well. But full-time jobs nowadays often require people to work up to 12–14 hours a day or 60–80 hours a week with no regular breaks for meals. Doctors on duty are expected to be on their feet more than 24 hours at a stretch, 2–3 times a week, and not fumble at work. In addition, each person is urged to exercise regularly, date and marry, have children and raise them well, be filial to parents, do voluntary work, and be involved in nation building during the remaining hours of the day. To accomplish all of these, more than 24 hours a day would be needed. However, it is argued that people who prioritise or manage time well and do quality stuff would still be able to find time to play golf, attend concerts, and go for holidays.

Monkey See, Monkey Do

There is a global culture of colonisation and cloning through international trade and information technology. Thus, from the monkeys of "see no evil, hear no evil, speak no evil", people have become "monkeys see, monkeys do". They learn to assert and sell themselves shamelessly or smartly at times. To succeed, there seems to be no place for honesty, humility, and modesty. They also adopt the same language and expressions; terminologies and titles; management and operations; franchises and lifestyles; idols and icons; diets and drinks; and diseases and disorders.

And when people sing "Count on me Singapore" in celebration each year, they also leave behind heaps of affluent litter as "one nation, one people" for others far away from their homes to clean up. Perhaps there is no alternative or choice in this "monkeys see, monkeys do" business. It has frequently been repeated that people are too dependent on those in authority. The likely truth is that these people have been too conditioned to obey instructions and follow directions in the mould of "monkeys see, monkeys do". Some "monkeys" keep setting new benchmarks for the rest with strained resources to chase and copy, often blindly or for the wrong reasons. Sadly, there is just no catching up. The standard bearers or trendsetters will always stay ahead.

"Monkey see, monkey do" also applies to following in the footsteps of uncompromising advocates of democracy, human rights, freedom of speech, and capitalism, which divides the world between extremes and perhaps introduces the new warfare of "state sans border".

Change, Choice, Control

Change is a fact of life, and so it is.

Change, such as the growth and development of a child and the four seasons, are part of nature. They may be anticipated with welcome. Natural disasters like earthquakes, floods, hurricanes and epidemic diseases are obviously destructive, traumatic, and feared, but there are also man-made changes that may be accidental, arbitrary, incidental, or intentional, such as industrial disasters, wars, terrorism, economic crises, or political upheavals.

Change may be a challenge to conquer and control or a fact of life for many.

When faced with change, a response is expected, and the response may be to avoid, ignore, adjust, or adapt to it. There is a choice, although effort is required. When change is threatening and coping efforts are exhausting, stress is felt. Such changes are usually imposed on the individual without choice. There may be arm twisting, blackmailing, or trading off involved.

Successful management of change presupposes choice and control. At a higher plane, it implies the power of politics, strength of forces, and reserve of wealth. In order to perpetuate control, the developed and powerful introduce constant changes such as IT, a knowledge-based economy, new policies, restructuring, merging, and recruitment of fresh personnel or talents.

Others become stressed because they are at the mercy of imposed changes that they have to keep catching up with to survive.

Through an understanding of human nature, marketing strategies, and forceful regulations, enormous amounts of money are amassed by enterprising innovators of fads and fashion and fanciful hardware and software upgrades. The manipulated consumers, who are enamored with choices for competitive products and hence slave in pursuit of brand names and latest gadgets, play an important role in enriching and supporting the quality lifestyles led by the developed and powerful.

Id, Change, Virtual Reality

In this era of globalisation, there is a relentless emphasis on "change" and thus there is an abundance of cliché statements on "change" (e.g., "change is the only certainty in life", "the only constant in life is change"). It is strange that in the midst of constant and continuous change, human nature has not changed (this is evidenced in the proliferation of rules and regulations, protocols and procedures, and laws and ethics to control and curb the complex and ingenious human commissions and omissions). Nevertheless, the need to change can be a matter of survival for individuals or society, so people have to be flexible and nimble, or innovative and entrepreneurial. On the other hand, there is also change for the sake of change, which becomes an end itself. Therefore, people in place must introduce continuous change to appear creative and progressive. Process supersedes product and results are inconsequential. In fact, it is difficult to assess or evaluate the outcomes of such change, because before the dust of change settles, another sweeper will come along. While high flying sweeping is commended, those on the ground have to continue inhaling the dust stirred up and get choked. When accounting and accountability are demanded, the virtual reality of "Enron Success" or "World-Com Connection" can be projected while rhetorical statements and white lies are employed. Losses in red become gains in black overnight through merging, restructuring, retrenchment, and selling of assets.

A virtual form of reality also exists in packaging, advertisement labels, restructuring and ISOs, JCI, SOPs on paper, measurement and manipulated statistics, relationships in name, title inflations, the free market, future trading, and paper assets. During rapid change, the vision and mission statements of yesterday become different from their translation and implementation today. There is a saying related to "word of honour" in Chinese that says "what is uttered cannot be retrieved by speedy horses". In the modern context of change, it seems what is uttered disappears into thin air.

One possible explanation for change and the power of change is the insatiable greed or need of the human id for immediate gratification and constant stimulation. From their experience and wisdom, our forefathers knew the id well. They cultivated the superego through upbringing to repress it and emphasised education of the ego to suppress it. Modern entrepreneurs also know the id well and they stoke it with fads, fashion, and fancies for commercial profits or economic gains.

Surrounded by all these changes, we need to strike an active balance of opposite virtues. We must not forget our vocational link to our patients when in pursuit of career advancement or market forces.

Secrets to Secular Success (and Power)

Make money by hook or by crook
Accumulate wealth beyond needs
Market consumerism as the global icon
Merge and restructure to compete and control
Optimise mastery, monopoly, and mass production
Negotiate with turn and twist to give little away
Interfere and destabilise, then exploit for gains
Sins are to be whitewashed for survival or success
Money is the alpha and omega

Courtesy, Civic Mindedness, Social Grace, Happiness

There are different perceptions on the regional or global ranking of courtesy, civic mindedness, social grace, and happiness. When high ranking is the result of spontaneous and genuine efforts, it reflects good mental health and cultivated lifestyle. But if it is achieved under duress, then mental health is likely to be at risk.

There could be a number of reasons for low ranking. The emphasis on "no free lunch" or "no one owes you a living" means that "everyone is on his own and for himself" or "I owe no one anything", which is the root of "kiasuism" and has been overused to describe almost everything but really means self-centredness and selfishness. Then there is the elitist top-down modelling effect. Superiority is endorsed, rank is right, money is king, title is queen, and bottom-up for the unselected is a futile struggle. The gap between the top 20% and the lower 20% widens and low ranking is the outcome, alongside the expression of displaced resentment or anger, ventilation of frustration, and plain "bochap" (who cares). Moreover, there is the prevalent habit of complaining against the backdrop of excellence and success constantly proclaimed. Complaining is safer than constructive criticism and serves as a way to cope with stress and for those with no say to say no. Finally, there are the unenlightened, antisocial, and mentally unwell groups that exist in every society.

Certification, Branding, and Franchises

Certification, branding, and franchises are big money-making businesses today. Without certification in areas of education, skill, performance, and product, one is handicapped in life. Therefore, entrepreneurs innovate and create ways and means of certifying others with qualifications and standards that are marketable. Life becomes a continuous pursuit of certification and re-certification. Many pay handsomely and willingly to be certified to enhance their market value. Others have no choice but to submit to the stressful process. Indeed, not all certifications guarantee quality and delivery. Only birth certificates and death certificates for all are not earned. But they too can be forged and used for different purposes.

Peddling Stress Management

In medicine, diagnosis is preferably made according to aetiology.
Treatment is then directed at removing the cause to allow natural healing.
When the cause is not understood or cannot be cured or controlled,
then treatment is symptomatic or management is palliative.
Modern stress management that earns big money is mostly symptomatic in approach.
There is little attention paid to the cause or stressor.

Often, the stressor is the management that creates unproductive stress.

(see Sloggers and Shirkers and History of Corporate Stress)

Stress management should therefore target both the stressed and the stressor.

Sadly, the peddler is often a helpless victim himself dishing out standard clichés.

Strange Outcome

Despite the crusading and championing of human rights and democracy, it has not produced an equal and egalitarian society. Instead, the gap between the rich and the poor and the haves and the have-nots has widened. Such is the power of predatory global corporate organisations; The engine of relentless competition and stress. Then there is the politically correct denial of differences in individual capability, capacity, and caprice that requires a differential, judicious, and enlightened approach instead of one size fits all.

The Mystery of Logic

To achieve quality of life, which includes better wage packages, There must be significant economic growth. To achieve sustainable economic growth, there has to be continuous restructuring, upgrading of skill, and increasing productivity. The price of quality of life is therefore relentless change, adaptation, and stress. However, upgrading of skill and increased productivity does not appear to apply to CEOs and directors of MNCs. The culture and operation of conglomeration is such that CEOs and directors are paid millions as an entitlement, even when the corporation is not making or even losing money. The lifestyle of entitlement seems to extend to the newer generations whose bread and butter are provided for by the labour of the older generation. Having their basic needs satisfied, they are no longer hungry to do any job. Pre-occupation with hedonistic pursuits replaces the drive to learn and improve. The id culture of constant stimulation and immediate gratification supersedes the superego culture of conscience and ideals. Meanwhile, the ego struggles to balance them with reality.

Needs, Wants, Technology, Business

Human needs of "yi 衣, shi 食, zhu 住, xing 行" are basic. When "clothes, food, dwelling, mobility" are satisfied, Fashionable clothing, gourmet and beverages, mansion living, automobiles, and jets are created. These new wants become new needs. Thereafter, needs and wants become intertwined in a continuous response. Technology is developed to be the answer and provider for constant stimulation and instant gratification. Technology in itself is neutral and good for progress and advancement. However, the hidden "intent" of competitive interests, business profits, and control of the market keeps spiralling in changes. Despite being satisfactory for use, products are constantly phased out by withdrawal of services and spare parts. New products are tweaked here and there and touted as desirable progress. In the process of consumerism and materialism, earthly resources are exploited, waste is created, and environments are destroyed. Man is pressured to learn, unlearn, and relearn in order to deliver. Those who are misfitting, unfit, and unwilling become unemployable and redundant as not everyone has the same capabilities. But man likes to think or believe that he has rights, freedom, and choice. In reality, he is also a slave to needs and wants and business greed. Not only is the population ageing, but the number of misfitting, unfit, and unwilling individuals are also growing. They feel deprived, frustrated, angry, and resentful. Mental and physical health becomes an issue and a burden. Technology creates new jobs but also destroys old jobs. Restructuring of the economy and upgrading of skills becomes a necessity. Meanwhile, partial solutions are found in foreign talents, computers, machines, and robots.

Checks and Balances

Democracy, human rights, and freedom of speech are not absolute.

It depends on who defines and decides.

When one's rights and freedom affect others', then it becomes relative.

Modern cultures and lifestyles encourage constant stimulation and instant gratification,

which breed addictive behaviour.

Boredom may lead people to seek stimulation and gratification that are harmful to the self and others.

Achievements and accomplishments in life require patience, perseverance, and passion.

Approach to Problems

What is the problem? (It is obvious that the problem must be identified.)

Whose problem is it? (Responsibility or liability is implied.)

Why is it a problem? (Question of circumstance or context.)

How to deal with the problem? (It depends on individual orientation.)

Orientation to the Problem

Philosophy	—	Altruism, Ideal, Pragmatism
Point of View	—	User, Provider, Purchaser, Payer, Politician
Purpose	—	Objective, Goal, Service …
Priority	—	Urgency, Agenda, Resources, Viewpoint again!
Professional	—	Expertise, Training, Practice, Territory
Progress	—	Evaluations — Not synonymous with New and Change, or Technology
Politics	—	To ensure continuation of power or popularity
Policy	—	Subject to Political, Economic, Social Forces
Payment	—	Funding, Reserves, Profits
Partnership	—	To Enhance Image and Competition, Inclusiveness
Propaganda	—	Mechanism to achieve covert/overt set goals
Prosecution	—	Medico-legal implication, Litigation, Boundary of Specialization, Insurance
Prevention	—	Predictable/Unpredictable accidents, events, incidents, scenarios, SOPs

The different orientations to deal with problems are not mutually exclusive. There is much overlapping, interplay, and compromise.

Healthy Person and Healthy Environment

It has been said that there is **no healthy person without a healthy environment**, and perhaps also vice versa. Thus, there are movements and organisations promoting healthy person-healthy environment projects and programmes. These would target:

Physical aspects — good housing and transport, clean air and water, supply of food and energy, hygienic environment, sewage and sanitation, control of pests and diseases, etc.

Social aspects — opportunity for education, fulfilling employment, fair income, religious freedom, racial harmony, law and order, justice, individual rights, space for recreation, healthy lifestyle, etc.

Psychological aspects — security, safety, stable and caring society, satisfying relationships at home, at work, and at play, etc.

These factors play important parts in both physical and mental health and are often taken for granted. Therefore, the clinical multidisciplinary team has an important role and function.

The government or society that provides a healthy environment and promotes healthy persons deserves as much credit as the physician, if not more.

Ecc. 1:9,11

What has been will be again
What has been done will be done again
There is nothing new under the sun
There is no remembrance of men of old
And even those who are yet to come
Will not be remembered by those who follow

10 Health Economics, Policy, and Manpower

Overview of Health Economics Issues

Healthcare cost is escalating worldwide.

Healthcare economics are complex, and one factor that contributes significantly to the **complexity** is that it has become a **commercial enterprise**.

Practice of medicine has changed from **one doctor** treating many patients at the primary care level to **many specialists and subspecialists** managing single patients at the secondary and tertiary levels. There is also a **proliferation** of **allied health professionals** or **workers**, **technicians**, and **managers**.

Developing society with limited resources provides **one size fits all** services that are **basic**.

With development and affluence, treatment or management becomes **individualised** or **customised**.

However, when society is developed and affluent and more resources are available, the **latest** investigations, machines, drugs, and procedures are introduced as necessary. It becomes the **new** baseline of **one size fits all** services that are **expensive** because of **new facilities** and **market forces** as well as **medico-legal issues** and **defensive practices**.

People are living longer and older with **chronic** and **degenerative diseases** that require long-term treatment and care. What is untreatable in the past is treatable now.

More diseases and disorders are added because of **new discoveries**, **changing concepts** and **thresholds**, and **medicalisation** of existential human imperfections and sufferings.

In addition, there is preventive **screening**, and **early** treatment, and **aesthetic medicine**.

Finally, we have so-called **lifestyle diseases** and **disorders** and **addictive** habits or behaviours.

Mental health, wellness, and **illness problems** are also gaining prominence and recognition.

The wise saying of "to cure sometimes, to care often, and to comfort always" becomes "to cure always, to care often, and to comfort sometimes."

Training of Future Psychiatrists

The training of future psychiatrists will be related to the training of future doctors.

The nature and purpose of medical education and training have been undergoing changes and are not static. Medical practice likewise undergoes changes for better or worse.

Medical schools have been revising their curricula, contents, directions, and emphases as well as tools and methods of teaching or training (e.g., problem- and team-based learning, virtual reality).

Based on growth of knowledge and advancement in management, there is a dilemma and tension in the balance of producing generalists or specialists at both the undergraduate and postgraduate levels. Years of medical courses and medical curricula vary. Levels of general competency and confidence also vary. The trend is towards life-long continuous medical education or professional development.

The **oath** and **pledge** we take are persons-centred, emphasising a compassionate approach to **cure**, **care**, and **comfort** for our patients and the special **fraternity** within the profession.

Declaration of Geneva [amended 68th WMA General Assembly, Chicago, USA in 2017]

["First" adopted by 2nd WMA General Assembly, Geneva, Switzerland, September 1948; amended by 22nd WMA, Sydney, 1968; 35th WMA, Venice, October 1983; 46th WMA General Assembly, Stockholm, September 1994; editorially revised by 170th WMA Council Session, Divonne-les-Bains, France, May 2005 and 173rd Council Session 2006]

AS A MEMBER OF THE MEDICAL PROFESSION:
I SOLEMNLY PLEDGE to dedicate my life to the service of humanity;
THE HEALTH AND WELL-BEING OF MY PATIENT will be my first consideration;
I WILL RESPECT the autonomy and dignity of my patient;
I WILL MAINTAIN the utmost respect for human life;
I WILL NOT PERMIT considerations of age, disease or disability, creed, ethnic origin, gender, nationality, political affiliation, race, sexual orientation, social standing or any other factor to intervene between my duty and my patient;
I WILL RESPECT the secrets that are confided in me, even after the patient has died;
I WILL PRACTICE my profession with conscience and dignity and in accordance with good medical practice;

I WILL FOSTER the honour and noble traditions of the medical profession;

I WILL GIVE to my teachers, colleagues, and students the respect and gratitude that is their due; [My colleagues will be my sisters and brothers (2006)].

I WILL SHARE my medical knowledge for the benefit of the patient and the advancement of healthcare;

I WILL TAKE PROMPT ACTION if patient safety is compromised from either internal physiological or external environmental causes;

I WILL ATTEND TO my own health, well-being, and abilities in order to provide care of the highest standard; [new]

I WILL NOT USE my medical knowledge to violate human rights and civil liberties, even under threat;

I MAKE THESE PROMISES solemnly, freely, and upon my honour.

But environmental and economic factors and administrative policies have made it difficult for our oath and pledge to be fulfilled.

These days, we do not have complete control over how we practise medicine. Administrators and management have the final say. **Clinical language and terminology are replaced by business terms such as:**

Corporatisation, CEO, case manager, case-mix, customer service, costing, packaging and marketing, health industry and clinical technology, entrepreneurial research, medical tourism, added value, KPI and performance bonus, and a host of other economic jargon.

Computerisation on the one hand facilitates management but on the other hand stifles flexibility and controls how procedures should be followed. There seems no place for altruism. Internet savvy consumers are no longer passive patients.

In training future psychiatrists, planners may consider the following:

What are the needs in terms of numbers and ratios?

This will depend on demographic changes, projections, and anticipated lifestyles, such as ageing populations, retirement, savings, family support, independent living, quality of life, substance abuse, etc.

One possible error in the projection of doctors needed and the capping of intake into medical school is the **one size fits all doctor to population ratio**. It was probably not taken into consideration that:

We are treating what have been considered untreatable.
We are treating more and more patients with chronic conditions.
We are treating more and more conditions for marginal benefit or improvement.
We are treating more and more people because of changing threshold criteria.
We are treating what others consider as "medicalisation" of problems in living and habits.
We are doing things for aesthetic or cosmetic reasons and the promotion of wellness.
Preventive screening and early intervention are promoted.
Finally, there is attrition due to migration, retirement, sickness, and death.

In the past, one doctor treated many patients (as whole persons), but now many doctors treat one patient (as divided parts).

How do we apportion our focus and development of resources to the:

> Primary healthcare level
> Secondary specialist level
> Tertiary super-specialist level
> Teaching, Training and Research level?

What do future psychiatrists need to know and how much and in what area?

We have been against the division of mind and body, but now we are dividing the "mind".

What are the territory or turf boundaries and medico-legal implications in practice?

Are we going to be DSM symptoms list checkers and persuaded to prescribe specific drugs approved by the FDA for specific diagnoses?

Will there be more demand for psychotherapy, medication, or genetic interventions?

What are the roles of future psychiatrists?:

> Is he going to be holistic and a team leader of other trained professionals?
> Is he going to retreat into the medical model of diseases, doing a nuts-and-bolts or assembly line job?

How is treatment or management going to be financed or paid?

In Singapore, we have Medisave, Medishield, Medifund, and other health insurance.

What do policymakers have in mind?

In some way, doctors contribute significantly to healthcare costs when they order expensive and advanced diagnostic investigations. Studies have shown that with good clinical history, well-trained doctors are able to correctly diagnose the majority of complaints (60–75%). Clinical skill in examination would add another 10–20% to confirm the diagnosis. Only a small portion of perhaps 5–10% would need special investigations.

Training Future Consultants

What matters most regardless of different postgraduate models and training programmes is to avoid **inbreeding** of **confusion** and **supposed experts** that lead to stagnation of progress.

Novices and trainees in psychiatry are struggling due to the confusion caused by **disparities** in clinical teaching and practice in terms of diagnosis and treatment. There are questionable didactic applications of certain diagnostic systems and algorithm prescriptions.

The nature of psychiatric illnesses or problems depends on the understanding or rationalisation of the **inter-relations, interaction**, and **integration** between the **individual** and his **environment**, between his **body** and **mind**, between the **neural circuits** and **mental functions**, and between his **present** and **past life events and experiences**. **Clinical conceptualisation** depends on the biological or psychosocial model employed. Although the current approach is **phenomenological**, it should not be synonymous with being **atheoretical**. The foundation of medicine is based on diagnosis and management according to

aetiology (i.e., **pathogenesis** and **pathophysiology**). Note what is **primary** or **secondary** in development.

When in training, one should have **curiosity** which is necessary for creativity, **diligence** which is necessary for achievement, and an **open mind** which is necessary for growth. Always ask to **clarify** or **verify** and try to **rationalise** what you do.

Learn as much as possible when you are young and inexperienced.

Learn from the **patient, family, and significant others**, and seek to **know** and **understand** them rather than just the **symptoms checklist, rating scales, MCQs**, and **OSCE**.

Because when you become a consultant, you may be **too proud** or **shy** to learn, and you will not be able to teach or avoid teaching what you do not know.

The worthy consultant should be **resourceful**, humble, and willing to learn.

The often quoted **Evidence-Based Medicine** is a **standardised** and **statistical** guide.

Its application is a bottom line **one size fits all** approach.

Advanced or improved management has to be **individualised** and **customised**, which calls for **personal experience** built up **rigourously** over the years.

Evidence-based medicine derives from **experience-based medicine** and complementary.

Beware of the persuasiveness of pharmaceuticals, which are driven by profits.

Classification of Mental Disorders is **atheoretical**, **syndromal**, and by **consensus inclusion**.

Not all mental disorders are **diagnosable** and they often are **forced into pigeon holes.**

Rigid adherence to ICD or the DSM leads to **thinking within the box** and **stagnation**.

Do not be complacent or smug just because it does not seem to matter whether a correct diagnosis is made or a proper treatment is given, or whether the patient may or may not respond, is unlikely to die, or does not complain, and no one is wiser.

To seek answers or solutions to problems, **clinical research** is necessary besides reading up. In randomised controlled trials, the larger the sample population and longer the duration of the study, the simpler the statistics will be and thus the more likely the validity and reliability of the findings. On the other hand, the smaller the sample size and the shorter the duration of the study, the more complex the statistics would be and the less likely the validity and reliability of the results.

Finally, experience and skill at the beginning are mostly acquired from subsidised patients. It should **benefit all** and not only later for those who can afford. We teach **"first do no harm"**, which is no harm to the body by what we do; no harm to the mind by what we say; and no harm to the pocket by what we charge. We need to ponder whether **our lifestyle** ought to be the **byproduct** of what we can manage or the **end-product** to achieve at all cost.

Science and Art of Medicine (various sources)

Treating the Bug that the Patient has is Science.
Treating the Patient who has the Bug is Art.
Therefore, treating the Disease is science and treating the Patient is Art.
To care with Competence is Science.
To care with Compassion is Art.

Best (unknown colleague)

In the best interest of the patient is not the same as giving our best.
Because our best may not be the best unless and until we become
the best.

First do no harm

No harm to the body by what we do
No harm to the mind by what we say
No harm to the pocket by what we charge

Cure, Care, Comfort

The wise physician teaches about
To cure sometimes, to care often, and to comfort always
Modern medicine and technology do the reverse
To comfort sometimes, to care often, and to cure always

Change and Human Nature

Change in life is said to be constant and continuous.
But the human nature of selfishness, greed, corruption, and cruelty
is unchanging.
In the race to create wealth, the environment is exploited, the
world is polluted by excess waste, and the climate is changing
which endangers all species, including human beings.
Hence the proliferations of rules and regulations, protocols and
procedures, and laws and ethics (but they are not universally
observed).
To control and curb the complex and ingenious human commissions and omissions.
Human behaviour is determined by biological instincts, social
influence, and legal control.
Foresight depends on hindsight; insight concludes "too little, too
late" because scenarios keep changing.

Digital Technology and Artificial Intelligence vs Knowledge and Belief and Human Response.

In data analytics, much depends on what is collated or downloaded and whether they are facts, fakes, or manipulated, such as in research and publications, marketing and profiteering, and policy mindsets.

It then depends on individual assessment, beliefs, and compliance with what is currently available, which may change and differ rapidly. Very often, knowledge and understanding do not ensure the appropriate action of complete adherence that is expected. Instructions and reminders may not be agreed upon and followed diligently.

Digital technology and AI do not seem to take into account human nature and quirks, individual experiences, personality traits, and prevailing mental states, such as anxiety, depression, paranoia, obsession, and perhaps "forgetfulness", all of which affect responses.

In medicine, particularly in psychiatry, the doctor needs to know his or her patient as a person and understand his or her nature of problems before giving opinions and advice, and should not simply follow AI algorithms by trial and error. Digital technology and AI do not replace the clinician who is guided by "first do no harm" and "to cure sometimes, to relieve often, and to comfort always".

Interestingly, St Paul in Roman 7:15, NIV said, "I do not understand what I do. For what I want to do I do not do, but what I hate I do."

Thus, although knowledge is power, it does not determine behaviour, which is influenced by biological instinct (the Id), psychosocial shaping (the Ego), and legal control (the Superego).

Covid-19 Impact On Mental Health And Illness

It is useful to be aware that Covid-19 is a "systemic" disease that could affect the body from "Head/(Brain) to Toes".

As such it could cause acute brain syndromes of confusion, disorientation, delirium and psychosis.

It could also lead to a whole host of mental disorders that is reactive and reactivating in nature.

It is useful to remember the general principles of the holistic biopsychosocial factors in predisposing, precipitating and perpetuating causative diagnoses and developmental dynamics.

It is also important to understand the inter-relation, interaction and integration of prevailing biopsychosocial factors in symptomatology or psychopathology.

When the brain is directly affected organic brain syndromes result. Depending on degree and severity and area involved psychiatric manifestations may arise e.g. encephalitis.

Majority of mental disorders would be "reactive in nature" which may be predisposing, precipitating and perpetuating.

"Reaction" may be due to the fear and stress of Covid -19 infection.

"Reaction" may be due to the direct infection of Covid-19 and the discomfort and side effects of treatment experienced.

"Reaction" may be due to the consequence of management and measures to control and contain the Covid-19 pandemic i.e. Circuit Breaker (CB)/Lockdown living, constant social distancing and personal hygiene.

During the circuit breaking family livelihood and individual relationships are affected. Hardship and deprivation emerge.

Personal dormant and latent issues may surface in friction and conflict, anger and abuse, frustration and fight.

Mental symptoms of anxiety, fear, stress, short term adjustment and long term adaptation of uncertain future would be common.

Depression of loss in normalcy, employment and income; isolation and loneliness might even lead to suicidal thoughts and behaviour.

Anxiety is the mother of psychopathology in predisposing, precipitating and perpetuating symptoms. Uncontrolled imagination could lead to delusional thinking and abnormal perceptions.

However, there are some positive aspects of the CB in bringing some families and communities closer, learning of sharing, kindly volunteerism, technology in communication.

Asymptomatic carriers are major worry and the hope is in the discovery of safe and effective vaccines and drug treatments for all.

Printed in the United States
by Baker & Taylor Publisher Services